MADELEINE

Losing a Soul Mate to Cancer

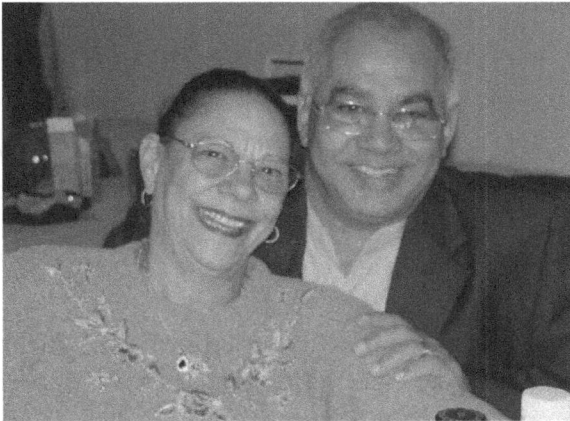

Clancy Philippe

Published by
Madeleine Philippe Cancer Foundation (Aus) Inc
http://www.mpcfaus.org

PO Box 8605
Carrum Downs, Vic 3201, Australia

clancy@cjp.net

Third Edition November 2014

Prologue

"When I play your song Meme*
the tears start rolling down my face...

I love you so much!

You have no idea how much we all miss you...

You put up the biggest fight of your life and
yet you stayed strong the whole time...

I had just started to build a
really good relationship with you!

I am going to cherish that for the rest of my life...

I will love you forever and always...

Always in me heart!

I miss you and love you so much...
You have no idea!"

:'(Molly Elise Tuplin-Kelly
(Granddaughter of Madeleine and Clancy)

*Madeleine Philippe

Introduction

This emotional rollercoaster describes the journey of one man losing his lifelong partner to cancer and details how he tries to come to terms with the bereavement and prepares to face life without her. It is an absorbing read, taking you right back to the early days of courtship and romance, and how the young couple married and moved from their native land in Mauritius to set up life in Australia. Cancer appears on the fringe of things with minor effect until Clancy's wife Madeleine is diagnosed with the disease herself. The couple's courageous ongoing battle over a number of years is detailed along with the emotional highs and lows many families face when dealing with this disease in their midst.

What makes this book stand out above others is that the author has with great openness, honesty and often raw intimate detail poured out his heart as he struggles in his efforts to save his wife from what turns out to be a terminal illness. After her passing, the reader is left feeling the emptiness, the loss and utter despair as if it was their own. The remainder of the story will surprise and provide plenty of food for thought. There are few authors who can in the simplicity of their writing make the words smile through the tears. A beautiful never ending love story, that shows great courage from both sides of the divide.

From the Author – Clancy Philippe:

This book began as a tribute to my late wife Madeleine whose five year battle with cancer opened the eyes of many to the tremendous strength and courage drawn from within the human spirit. The loss of my wife, best friend and soul mate has left a void in my life that will never be filled. However, in writing this book, I have found clarity from the confusion and a reason to live again. Certain events occurring subsequent to Madeleine's departure have altered my whole attitude towards life, death and the immortal soul within us. In writing this book, I want to share our story with others so that they too may find hope and courage in their own journeys.

Three years on since the passing of Madeleine, I am still very much in love with her. Our love for each other is growing stronger and I feel that she is still around. Cooking her recipes is now therapy for me and whenever I am cooking, it's like some form of spiritual re-connection.

The proceeds from the publication of this book will be donated to the Madeleine Philippe Cancer Foundation (Aus) Inc.

Dedication

This book is dedicated first and foremost to Madeleine, the *'Love of my Life'*. She meant everything to me. She was the best wife, friend, mother, grandmother and mother in law that God ever put on this earth.

She made my life complete and I am forever thankful for that. To be blessed with her unconditional love and presence throughout thirty four wonderful years of married life has been an honour and a privilege. She will continue to be my Soul Mate throughout eternity – not even cancer can take her away from me.

I also dedicate this book to the loved ones, family and real friends who stuck by me before, during and after our five year battle with cancer - I love you from the bottom of my heart. Without this support, I do not think that I would have survived and lived to tell the tale. In particular, I wish to make a special mention for the first of her generation, great granddaughter Lilly Madeleine Adams. It was a blessing for me to have her named after Madeleine.

My dedication is also directed to Dr. Ian Haines and his team at Cabrini Hospital. They provided incredible support to Madeleine and myself. They lightened the load, fended off cancer as best they could and offered hope when there was none. Thank you on behalf of the family.

I must also not forget the loved ones, friends and Madeleine's fans scattered all over the globe, offering incredible support and comfort when the going got tough, and through their *'collective prayers'* made it easier on Madeleine and myself, during these difficult times.

Acknowledgements

Madeleine and I wanted to write a book together and share our experience in the fight against cancer in the hope that our journey would help others in the same situation. Unfortunately, cancer took Madeleine away before a single word was written. However, that has not stopped her from having her say and throughout the entire book she has been its inspiration and guide. She is still very present in my life.

To my principal editor, Liz Coates - thank you for your skills and friendship. Your honest and helpful comments ensured that I did not wander too far from the facts. There were many times when my 'emotionally charged' writing strayed a little, but you helped me see through the tears and enabled me to reveal my beliefs and innermost feelings. You certainly rescued me from many embarrassing mistakes and came at a time when I was struggling for words.

Amongst the other people who have helped with the production of this book, I wish to name the following: Farouk Sohawon for his wonderful advice, Annabelle Adams for her intuitive recommendations on the front and back cover designs, Yolanda Aquino for her advice on the title for the book and Gerard deBaize, Norman Coates and others who have acted as draft readers and offered their invaluable input. Also, I wish to thank Michael Barbato, Elizabeth Ducasse, Lindsay Noë, Irlande Alfred, Chin, Patrick Morel, Lucas Sikiotis and Mary Dallas for their timely interventions that put faith back into people. A special thank you to Henri Maurel for the creation of a special dish 'Saumon Maddy – Saveur des Îles' dedicated to Madeleine and to Michael Barbato, author of 'Reflections of a Setting Sun' and Kate Legge of 'The Australian' newspaper for their permission to reproduce some of their writings. I wish to thank the City of Greater Dandenong for their wonderful support that enabled me to care for Madeleine in the best possible manner. My sincere apology goes to others I may have missed.

It would be remiss of me not to mention the love and affection of family and loved ones who never stopped supporting Madeleine and I through our five year battle with breast and ovarian cancers. Their continuing support since Madeleine's passing has been immeasurable. From deep within my soul, I say thank you on behalf of both of us.

Last but not least, I wish to acknowledge all the family and friends who never lost faith in me, urging me to carry on and accomplish what many thought was going to be an impossible task.

Pouring out my emotions into writing whilst in the grips of the utmost pain and grief after losing Madeleine, has been the hardest project that I have ever attempted in my life. The box of tissues has been my closest companion throughout the composition of this book - it still is.

Table of Contents:

Chapter 1

The Beginning of the End

Ward 3 South, Cabrini Hospital, Malvern in Melbourne, Wednesday February 9, 2011

At 8.30 am, I grabbed my mobile phone and wrote the following:

"I am currently in Madeleine's hospital room watching her slowly fade away. She has lost the will to fight and is slipping away fast. The doctor has advised that it is only a matter of time. I am just devastated to find that such a lovely and caring human being has been almost totally consumed by this dreadful disease. She is now on morphine to ease the pain.

I don't know what more to say. I will keep you posted and give you a call when things settle down. I am seeing the doctor tomorrow re: path from here.

Clancy"

I was watching Madeleine, my beloved wife of thirty four years, in a semi-comatic state and awaiting the inevitable.

Cancer was not something that other people had. It was very much with us.

We had tried every possible avenue to conquer that dreadful disease. Madeleine's body had been battered, injected with cytotoxic chemicals and exposed to radioactive radiation hoping that the malignant cancer tumours would die and stop interfering with her bodily functions.

Suddenly, she regained consciousness, opened her eyes, reached for me, looked me in the eyes and said: "Aide moi?" (Help me?) Those two words broke my heart beyond repair.

Real words of comfort could not come out of my mouth. I had no words to say because there was nothing that I could do to help her. There was nothing that the best doctors or even the best hospitals in the whole world could do. My heart was imploding inside my chest. I could not breathe. My whole world was empty and my loving partner, best friend and Soul Mate was leaving me. She was saying *"Good Bye"*. I could see that in her eyes. The same loving eyes that *"talked to me and loved me without the need for words"* were now filled with despair. The same hands that had been so loving and had done so much for me, had become almost motionless.

Why Madeleine? Why me? What did we do to deserve this fate? Madeleine and I had always been one. Yet, half of me was being wrenched away. Wherever she was going, I was going too. My Louloune*, this just cannot be true. I must be dreaming. A bad dream that has no ending.

* Madeleine's nickname

I was numbed. Tears were running down my cheeks. I became oblivious to the outside world and could not help but travel back in time to the moment when I first set eyes on that beautiful and passionate woman, some thirty six years ago.............

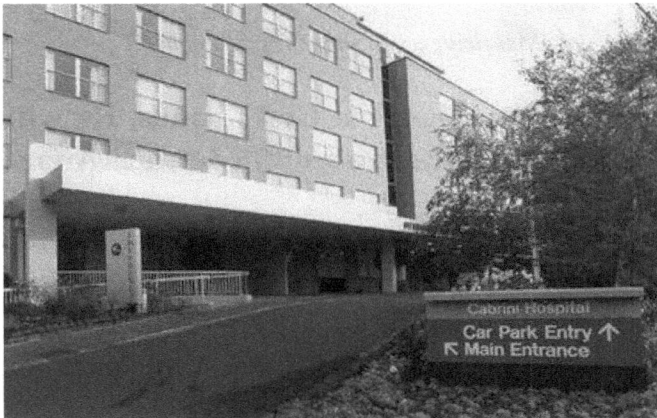

Cabrini Hospital, Malvern, Melbourne

Chapter 2

She was my Cleopatra

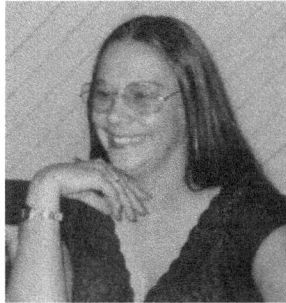

Madeleine when she captured my heart

"If you placed your heart in God's hands, He will place your heart in the hands of a worthy person." Anon

I remember meeting Madeleine for the first time. It was on August 1, 1975 at 9.00 am in the Town Clerk's office at the Municipality of Curepipe in Curepipe, Mauritius. I was taking up my appointment with the Municipal Council of Curepipe as Town Engineer.

I was in the Town Clerk's office when a person with an incredible presence, walked in to introduce the new Town Librarian who was also starting on the same day.

That person was Madeleine and I could not keep my eyes off her. She was wearing a Scottish kilt pattern skirt and coat, with a yellow blouse. I was then 26 years old and she did something to me - not quite love at first sight, but she was definitely someone who struck a chord in me.

I settled into my new position and for some reason enjoyed her company whenever she came into the main office. She told me some time later that she had noticed how I always found some good excuse to have a chat with her.

She was one of those people who socialised well and was way ahead of her time in that she had an openness of mind that challenged some of the 'good old days' thinking. Her best friends were male rather than female. She had just been through a divorce and was left to fare on her own with two boys aged 11 and 12 years old. Her pay was not that generous and she was battling with bills and rent to pay. Nevertheless, she found ways to stretch the budget and looked after her home and sons very well. Her house was always immaculately kept and everybody found a welcome there. When she discovered I had nowhere to go between normal working hours and attending council meetings at the Curepipe Town Hall, she offered me an open invitation to come and have coffee at her place after work instead of being on my own.

I jumped at the opportunity and got to know her better. I walked in one evening after a football match covered in mud and asked if I could have a shower at her place. Those days changing rooms were a rare thing at football training venues. She initially looked at me in disbelief, smiled and then said OK.

I found that she was a woman of incredible intelligence, charm and personality. She was very active within the community and President of the Cercle de Curepipe. This establishment was one of the high profile social clubs in town.

She had a touch of class that showed through in her elegant demeanour and yet simple approach to life. I could not help saying to myself that she was someone special, the kind of person you rarely came across. She had obviously been well brought up and educated. Her manners were impeccable and she was always simply, yet elegantly dressed.

She had a very strong, yet very pleasant personality – always commanding respect without appearing overbearing. Her presence was very much welcomed by one and all, in that she would actively and positively contribute to her social environment. It was something that stayed with her all through her life.

Once you meet her, you would never forget her. She was a joy to be with. She was a true friend who was not scared to express her thoughts and feelings. She had an entourage that had enormous respect for her and I really felt privileged to have become part of that. More so, her close friends felt that our developing relationship had something very unique and deserving. She had just been through and was still going through very tough times. She needed someone in her life who really cared - then I came along. Two people could not have cared better for each other.

Our love for each other blossomed and it was very evident that we paired so well together, complementing each other in many ways. I was what I would call very 'bachelor boy' in my approach to life at the time and was not actively looking for a girl friend or partner. Yet, I strongly felt that she was someone that I could spend the rest of my life with. It just happened, the chemistry was right.

No adjustment in our individual lives was necessary. We were like pieces of a jigsaw puzzle slotting together to become one. We belonged to each other and accommodated each other in a way that made it inevitable that we were destined to be together forever.

One of her most obvious attributes, which made life very enjoyable for many, was her love for cooking.

She would create dishes that had her special signature and left invitees to her table yearning for more. I was no exception. At the time, I could not even cook an egg let alone some of the more complex dishes I had started to enjoy. Her culinary skills were complemented with impeccable table manners.

She was someone you would be very proud to be with at any social gathering. She could talk to anyone whether they were down and out or public figures. She was equally at ease with everyone. She shone at high society gatherings by displaying her impeccable savoir faire. I understand that her mother Thérèse was very particular in the upbringing of her children. She brought up her kids the old fashioned way with particular attention to their education, social skills and knowledge of the arts.

One night, I attended a club dance at the Cercle de Beau Bassin with my cousins and Madeleine was there representing the Cercle de Curepipe at the dance. She had at the time a flowing mane of hair that befitted her image. She looked stunning - almost Cleopatra like. I fell in love with her that night.

We were invited back to her place after the dance to savour her famous Saturday night vegetable and oxtail soup. I was in the back seat of the car with her and gave her what must have been the longest kiss on record.

For those of you who know Curepipe, the kiss started at Eau Coulée and lasted until Ste Thérèse Church (some 3 km in between). Madeleine later told me she was surprised she had not passed out. That night, I did not go home and to say the least we had a very passionate night.

We started going out together and all hell broke loose when people found out that one of the most eligible bachelors in town was going out with a divorcee. Those days a divorcee was some sort of pariah and suddenly Madeleine and I were the talk of the town. Discussions as to how to stop this affair were even held at the highest level among the Councillors. At work, a fellow head of department at the Council was approached by the powers that be and was asked to talk me out of this relationship. He declined by saying that we were both unattached and he did not see anything wrong in what we were doing. Well meaning colleagues apparently met in private and also discussed various options to talk me out of this affair. They even considered approaching my parents to warn them of this impending inappropriate relationship. Prospective fathers in law, who had considered me a good catch for their daughters, added fire to the situation by further fuelling the debate. Within the family, the rumour mill was working overtime.

I just ignored all this and went on my merry way. In my heart, I knew for sure that I was doing the right thing. I remember an uncle who had the utmost respect for me saying at the time: *"Given your high standing in the community and the respect that everybody has for you, you can afford to ignore all this. People in the end will respect your decision."* They did and our relationship was later dubbed by many as a real 'Love Story'. Madeleine certainly did not let them down. Our relationship flourished a thousand fold instead.

My parents first heard about the affair from unknown sources and initially expected the romance to be short lived. However, when they heard positive reports about Madeleine, who was then Deputy Librarian at the Curepipe Carnegie Library, they soon changed their minds. Sadly, my Dad never got to meet her. He died the same night he had arranged a get together to welcome her to the family.

Madeleine did not escape the gossip mongers and the scourge of public opinion either and was subjected to bullying because of female jealousy arising from her going out with me. We held firm and did not allow these events to stop us from spending time together.

On this note, I should mention that Madeleine did have concerns about the effect our continuing relationship would have on me.

When I asked her to become my beloved wife, her first concern was for me and what I was letting myself in for. Her consideration for others (in this case me) took priority over her own interests. She sat me down and laid all her cards on the table knowing this could be to her own detriment.

She told me that she was 8 years older than me, a divorcee, had 2 boys and that because of my position as Town Engineer, marrying a divorcee was not the right thing to do. I told her that all this did not worry me in the least and that I was very intent in marrying her. I found out later that she obtained the consent of her two boys before accepting to become my darling wife. In Curepipe, the breaking news was all about this 'Love Story' of the time. They were not wrong, it was indeed the 'Love Story' of a lifetime. We were married on May 2, 1977 and celebrated at a delightful function at the Port Louis Tennis Club. It was later reported that almost everybody was a bit, if not very tipsy that night.

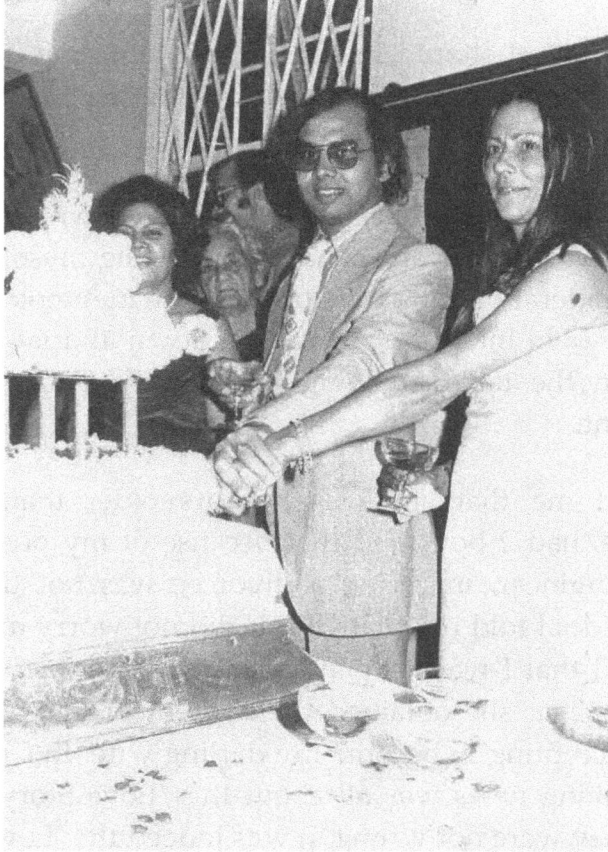

Our wedding at the Port Louis Tennis Club

As newlyweds, we went back to our place, rather Madeleine's, for the night before spending two weeks at the Trou aux Biches seaside resort. In the morning, a friend of ours dropped in to see us before we left and she said: *"How was it last night?"* Madeleine answered: *"Am still a virgin as he was too drunk and fell asleep!"*

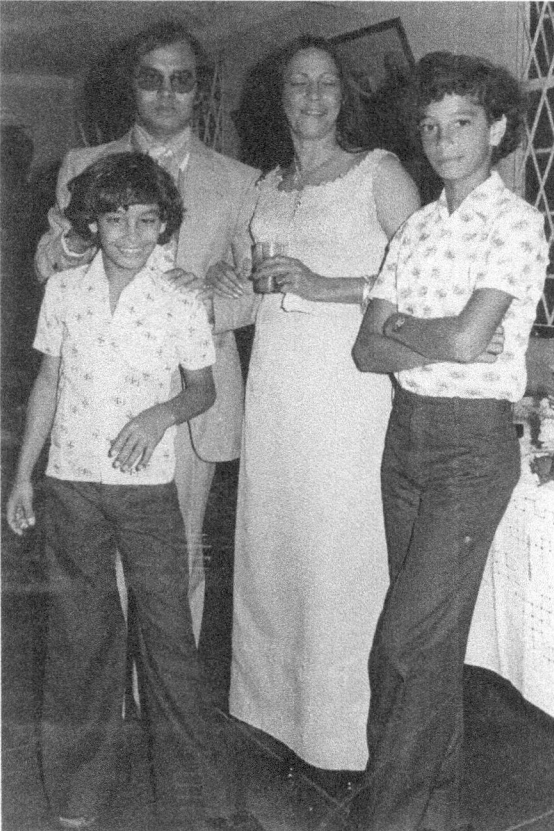

Madeleine, Clancy, Gerard & Michel

The last thing I remembered was having the two boys in my arms for a cuddle. However, we made up for it when we were at the seaside bungalow in Trou aux Biches where we had a wonderful honeymoon.

I was also in no doubt whatsoever that I had found that special person with whom I would spend the rest of my life. She was indeed special, really special.

Chapter 3

The Early Years with Cancer in the Family

"Life is about experiencing. Experiencing not only happy times but also sad times." Anon

We settled in as husband and wife in Curepipe, with the two boys. Madeleine by then had been appointed Librarian of the Carnegie Library. Our lives revolved around the family, friends and work. Life at home was pretty hectic with visitors coming in almost daily and most weekends were taken up with some family or friends get together. Madeleine's cooking attracted visitors and there was always enough food to accommodate one or two more guests. For more, a little bit of creative cooking converted dinner for six into dinner for twelve. The Auleebux brothers, who were both confirmed bachelors, dropped in almost daily for a drink and invariably for a nice dinner. We also had the house renovated with the addition of another lounge area and patio. Life was good and could not have been better. My brother Josian who also worked in Curepipe regularly dropped in for lunch with us.

There were card games that my mother Daisy, brother Josian, Grandmother Emilie and others would enjoy on a regular basis. Madeleine always made sure that when she was home, there would be special treats for the week end meals. Gol Auleebux was a fine gourmet and many discussions were held on the best techniques to extract the best flavours and results from ingredients. Madeleine was renowned for her culinary skills and that got me into trouble one day. She prepared a venison curry with embrevade beans on rice. That dish was so good that I could not help saying: *"Someone could marry you just for your food."* Madeleine responded by saying: *"So you married me for my cooking."*

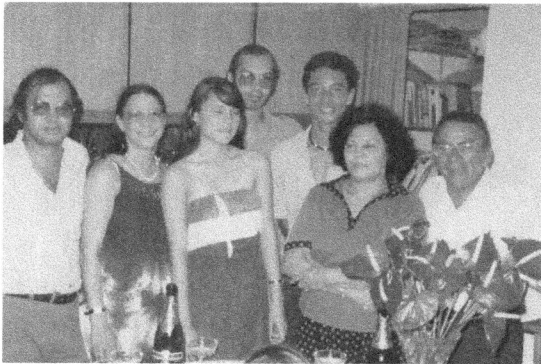

From left to right Clancy, Madeleine, Lilette (sister in law),
Josian (Clancy's brother), Gerard (son), Daisy (Clancy's mother)
and Marcel (Madeleine's father)

Madeleine's father Marcel who was still in Mauritius, regularly joined us at work on Fridays and we would take him home to spend the weekend with us. The kids would have great fun teasing their grandfather. He used to drive Madeleine berserk with advice as to the best way to cook certain dishes. On one occasion he asked Madeleine to put one extra ingredient in a dish that she was preparing. Madeleine ignored the request. When the meal was served he said: *"It's good that you listened to me, I can taste the difference."*

Madeleine and I were always together, and were seen travelling together at all times. The two of us had become one. Gol Auleebux always said that we complemented each other and that our marriage was a match made in heaven. Unfortunately, Madeleine had multiple miscarriages and for health reasons we gave up trying to have more children. We already had two boys and they kept me busy enough coping with their 'mischiefs'.

Since the 1950's and after independence in 1967, many Mauritians left Mauritius for Australia in search of a better future. Madeleine had three brothers and a sister there whilst I also had numerous relatives who had been part of this big migration. I learnt a lot about Madeleine's side of the family. She told me about how she lost her mother to breast and ovarian cancer.

In 1978, we learnt that Madeleine's sister Michèle who was in Melbourne had successfully battled ovarian cancer after surgery and chemotherapy.

In 1979, we decided to visit the family in Australia and see for ourselves why people called it the 'lucky country'. Australia was such an eye opener we could hardly wait to get back to Mauritius, so we could apply for our migration permit to join them.

We eventually migrated to Australia in June 1982. Madeleine's sister Michèle had asked that we settle in Sydney to be near her. Around the same time, Michèle had a cancer flare up and was undergoing chemotherapy again for ovarian cancer. Whether it was by choice or coincidence, not much was said about the cancer flare up at this time despite its seriousness. Even Madeleine's brother Guyto had moved from Melbourne to Sydney to be near her.

There was an economic downturn at the time and work was difficult to find. After spending nine months unsuccessfully looking for work in Sydney, I took up a position with the Mildura Shire Council in the State of Victoria. Until the job offer was made, I hadn't a clue where Mildura was! Mildura is located some 800 kilometres from Sydney in the North West corner of the

State of Victoria, bordering New South Wales and South Australia respectively.

We were living out of suitcases from one home to another. These nine months were hard but happy. Throughout it all, Madeleine never once complained. She did however express a feeling of guilt at one point, telling me that I had given up a very good job in Mauritius for unemployment in Australia. Madeleine also became pregnant but lost the baby.

Madeleine was happy in that she would have a home that she could call her own again. We had rented a house in Mildura over the telephone and expected that as it was in the centre of town, it would be OK. We travelled all night and arrived in Mildura on a Friday morning. Much to our horror, our new home was sited between office buildings with their walls only six inches from the house windows. The house itself was old, dark and decrepit with worn, patched-up carpets. The absence of any natural light made the house feel depressing and unwelcoming. Madeleine had a look inside and said to me: *"I am not staying here, take me back to Sydney."* We spent the rest of the day visiting real estate agents and just could not find a place to rent. We moved into hotel accommodation and stayed there for seven weeks, until we moved into an apartment not far from work.

Until we moved into the apartment, we were eating regularly at the famous Mildura Workingmen's Club.

Whilst I was at work, Madeleine would keep busy by visiting the town and Mildura's tourist attractions. She would also spend time doing her favourite pastimes, crosswords and jigsaw puzzles or reading novels.

We moved into the apartment with no furniture as our household goods were in transit in Sydney, waiting to be trucked to Mildura. We bought one bed, a table and four chairs, two dishes, two sets of cutlery, basic kitchen utensils and a good knife. A good knife is always important when preparing ingredients for cooking. Madeleine had a home that she could her own again. She was very relieved and was able to spend lots of time in the kitchen. Although we lived a very modest and spartan life in Mildura for five years, we had the best years of our lives together here, getting to know each other really well.

Michel our son had a job as apprentice turner and fitter in Sydney. Gerard joined the Australian army. I had the challenge of adapting to Local Government in Victoria. At that time in Australia, one had to be a registered municipal engineer to be appointed either municipal engineer or deputy municipal engineer.

I was advised to undertake studies in municipal engineering to meet these demands. In Mildura, apart from rare visits from relatives from Melbourne and Sydney, we were pretty isolated. Friends were few and far between. I was studying by correspondence which meant all my free time was pretty much used up. Besides, the people we knew in Mildura had their own problems to worry about. Nevertheless, Madeleine and I spent many memorable moments fishing and picnicking on the banks of the Murray River. Once you enjoy the Murray River, it gets in to your blood and becomes part of you. Those Murray River days filled us with happy memories.

You may recall that Madeleine's sister Michèle had undergone chemotherapy in 1978 for ovarian and bowel cancers. We stayed with her in Sydney when we first arrived in Australia. The bowel and ovarian cancers metastasised in early 1984. Madeleine commuted between Mildura and Sydney to look after Michèle in conjunction with her brother Guyto. I stayed in Mildura to work and Madeleine would come back every fortnight by coach travel to do the cooking and washing and to make sure that I was OK.

I was glad that Madeleine got to spend quality time with her sister whom she loved very much. Along with her brother Guyto, Madeleine offered invaluable support to Michèle during these difficult times.

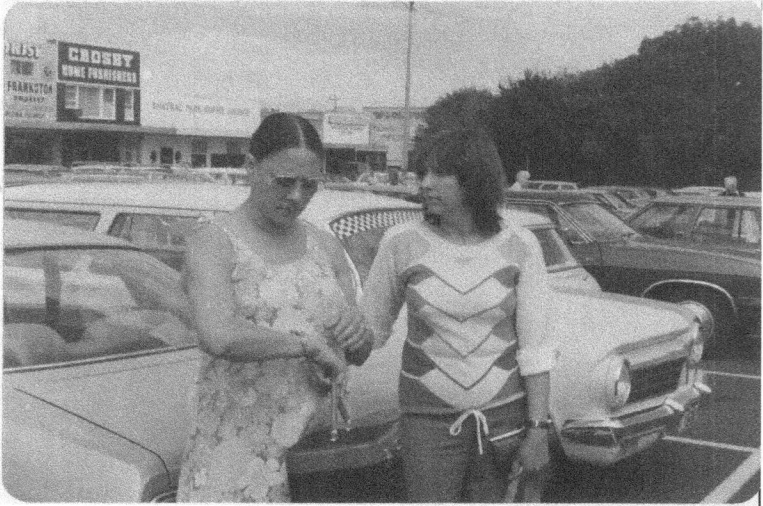

Madeleine and sister Michèle

On March 31, 1984 I received a phone call from Madeleine telling me it was over. Her sister had passed away after courageously battling this dreadful disease. I still remember Michèle's happy disposition when I visited her in hospital, despite knowing that it was only a matter of time. I saw for the first time how cancer could almost totally consume a very beautiful and caring person. She was only 44 years old then.

Madeleine was badly affected by the loss of her only sister. Michèle and I had got to know each other very well over the years and I loved her very much. She was so happy that Madeleine had met me and that we had such a great marriage. She and Madeleine were very alike.

During one of their intimate sisterly conversations Michèle told Madeleine: *"You have a very good husband. Enjoy life for tomorrow does not belong to us"*.

On Michèle's birthday every year, Madeleine would suffer some sort of mini depression. She lost her mother Thérèse under similar circumstances aged 50 years old.

In 1987 we celebrated my qualification as a registered municipal engineer in Victoria. Our sacrifice paid off almost immediately when I was appointed Deputy Shire Engineer at the Shire of Rosedale in Central Gippsland, State of Victoria. The memorable times we had in Mildura were about to be surpassed by our stay in Rosedale. In March 1988, we celebrated Madeleine's 50th birthday in style. The whole family turned up from Sydney and Melbourne and the local hotel was fully booked for the occasion. Our Rosedale friends and the family had a superb night and Madeleine had a 50th birthday celebration to remember.

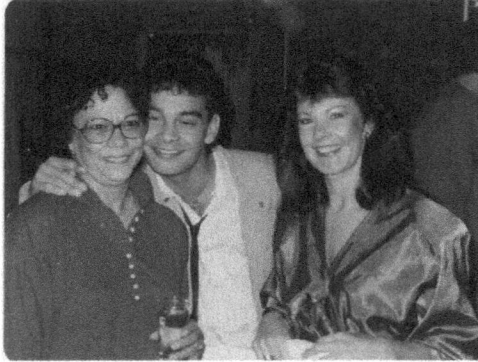

Madeleine's 50th birthday, with Michel (son) and friend Lee

The same year, we celebrated the birth of our first grandchild, Annabelle who was born in Sydney on October 24, 1988 with Madeleine there for her birth.

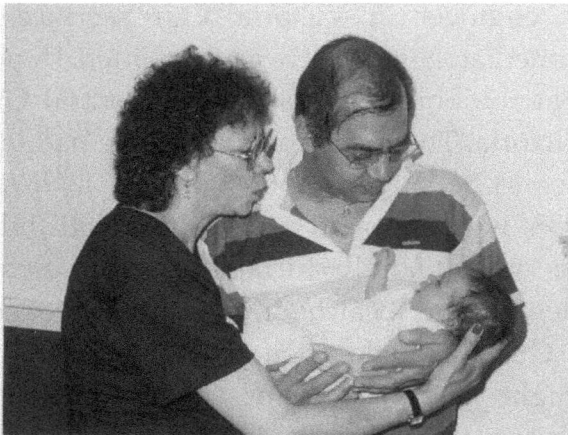

Madeleine and Clancy with Annabelle

Three months later we were both in Sydney to attend her christening. We returned to Rosedale from the christening with three months old Annabelle. Her parents were staying at the in-laws and had difficulties in coping with her. Whilst we were saying good bye, Annabelle's mum Chimène said: *"Take her with you"*. Dad Michel said: *"Yes!"* Madeleine said: *"What!"* We took baby Annabelle with us and I recall the trip down from Sydney to Rosedale like yesterday. The air conditioning in the car broke down and it was a hot summer. We had to stop every two hours to take care of the little one.

At 51, Madeleine was back to washing nappies and looking after a three months old baby. We were nevertheless very happy to have her with us and everybody in Rosedale knew her. *'Annabelle became the daughter we had always wished for.'* Annabelle learnt to walk, talk and do all the other interesting things that babies do with us. She also won the hearts of all the Council employees at the Rosedale Shire Council. She was always first through the door, rushing into the Council offices and asking for her Gpa. The interesting coincidence was that Madeleine used to visit her mother at the Curepipe Town Council and the staff all knew her there.

Life in Rosedale suited Madeleine perfectly. The Rosedale Township is the sort of perfect place where you are far enough from the city rush, but near enough to Melbourne when we had to visit relatives and friends or do some shopping for our Mauritian cuisine. We spent lots of time together in the garden and in 1992, Madeleine won the prize for the best garden in town.

However, cancer was to strike again. My mother Daisy who stayed alternatively between my brother Josian and myself, died on December 5, 1991 from pancreatic cancer. She had been admitted to Sale hospital and Madeleine commuted daily between Rosedale and Sale to be by her bedside during the day and offer her support. Josian or I stayed with her at night time as things went from bad to worse.

Madeleine also cooked her lunch and dinner daily as she could not cope with hospital food. This dedication to others is a perfect illustration of Madeleine's way of caring for others.

In 1992, I was appointed Shire Engineer. We moved into the Council Shire Engineer's house where we had numerous parties and get togethers. It was, to say the least, a real mansion and had three spare rooms and multiple bathrooms besides our own. There was plenty of extra accommodation for our town dweller relatives and friends who regularly came to our place in Rosedale to regenerate and have a break from the hurly burly of Melbourne or Sydney. These days were, by far, the very best we had together in that we spent so much time and did so many things together. Whether it was the countryside setting or something else, the romantic times were often and many. I recall with pleasure the times when lunch time resulted in me returning to work late. Today, this sort of impromptu romance just does not happen. We are all too busy chasing our tails.

In 1994, following Local Government reform in the State of Victoria, I was made redundant. We moved to Melbourne and bought a house in Carrum Downs, Melbourne. Madeleine (Meme to the grandchildren) and I had been missing the grandchildren and family in Melbourne and felt this move would bring us closer together. By then, the family had grown and in addition to Annabelle, we had another granddaughter Jennifer born in 1991 and grandson Nicholas born in 1993.

We also celebrated the births of our twin grandsons Brandon and Joshua in 1996 and a year later celebrated our 20th wedding anniversary.

We moved into our new house and Madeleine was very happy. Needless to say our front door was like a revolving carousel with visitors and guests coming and going regularly. One of the main attractions was Madeleine's cuisine.

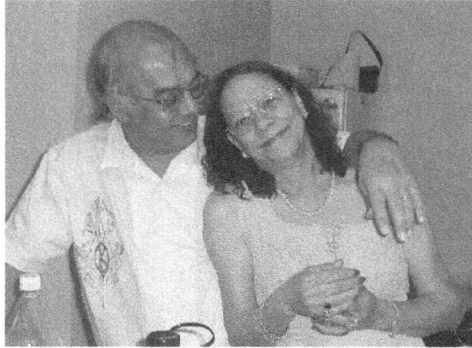

Our 20th wedding anniversary, wearing her wedding dress

This combination of my engineering background and Madeleine's culinary instinct led us to experiment on very diverse styles of cuisine. We concocted sausages, pies, pastas, exotic curries sourced from Maharajah recipes, dim sims, soups, breads, cakes, smoked meats, tripled cooked meats, rotis, stir fried Chinese dishes, slow cooked rich red and white wine marinated French casseroles, steamed pastries, Mauritian and Malagasy bouillons, rich game fares and many more.

We also became very involved in community activities and about the same time, we established the *'Mauritius Australia Connection'* web site, incorporating the *'Recipes from Mauritius'* web site.

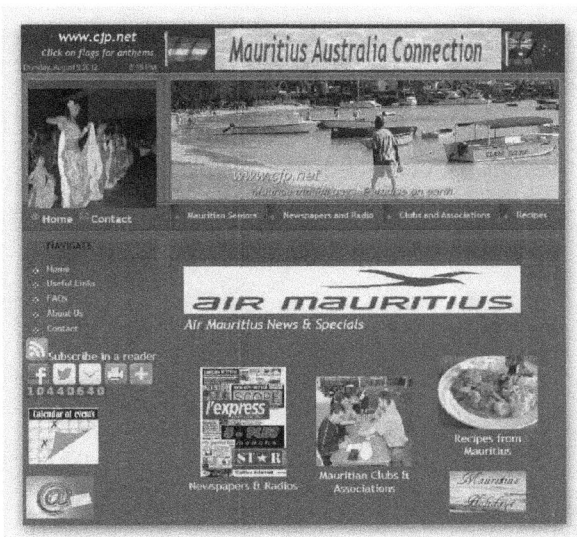

Mauritius Australia Connection web site

This was a landmark achievement at the time as unbeknown to us we had set up the very first web sites promoting Mauritius and its cuisine on the world wide web.

We also co-wrote articles for the media, in newspapers such as the Chicago Tribune and web blogs.

The Lonely Planet Travel Guide commissioned us to write the food and drinks section in their Travel Guide to Mauritius, Rodrigues, Reunion and Seychelles.

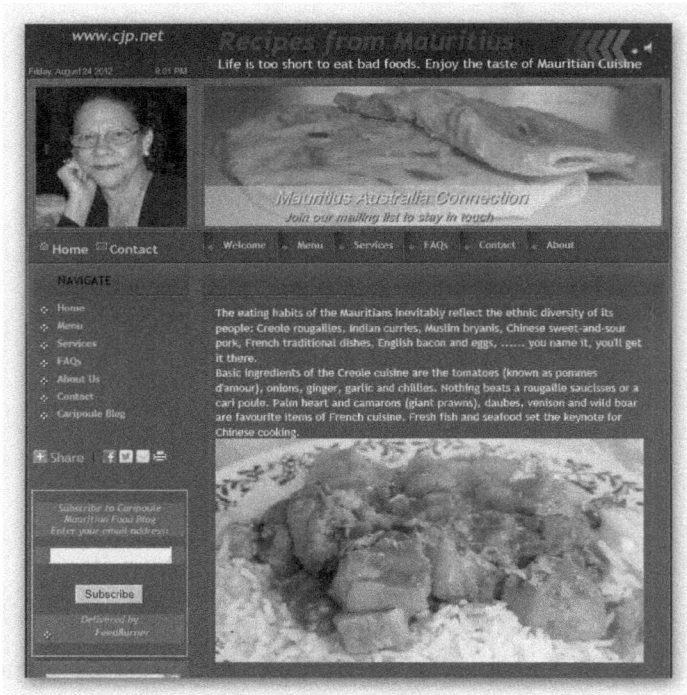

Recipes from Mauritius web site

I researched the cuisines, experimented and Madeleine would support with her culinary 'savoir faire'. Madeleine had this innate ability to taste any food and tell you which ingredients had been used in its preparation. Our stay in the winemaking region of Mildura complemented our knowledge of the edible, with an appreciation of wines and their pairing with foods.

In the same vein, Madeleine knew her Scotch whiskies and many restaurants were challenged when they substituted their drinks.

Life was really exciting and we left no 'stones unturned' in the undertaking of any projects that we would identify as worth doing. Madeleine was just as keen as me in exploring new ideas, especially in her passion for cooking.

Chapter 4

Breast Cancer makes its appearance

"A man truly loves you when missing you is his hobby, caring for you is his job, making you happy is his duty, and loving you is his life." Anon

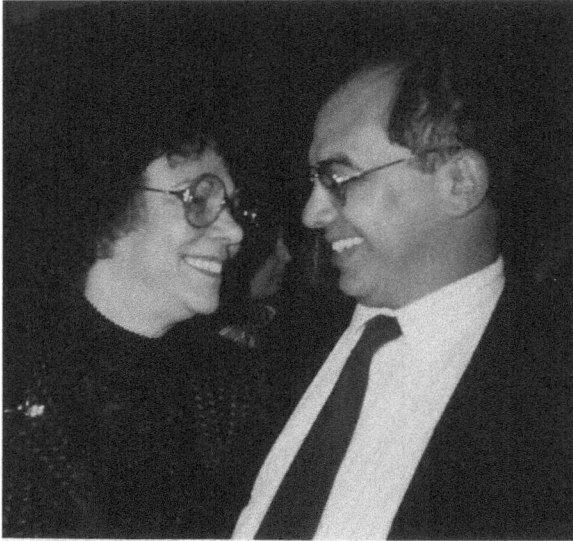

Happy Madeleine and Clancy

We settled in Carrum Downs. After a stint as an engineering consultant on local government asset management, I took a new job at the Australian Road Research Board in Vermont South, Melbourne assisting Local Government in Australia with road engineering research. One of the responsibilities of the position was to liaise with Local Government authorities and to meet with Council engineers across the whole of Australia. At the same time, I represented Local Government road engineering research on the peak body of the Institution of Engineers Australia which also meant having to attend National Conferences on Local Government Engineering in all states. Madeleine accompanied me on all these visits and we had the time of our lives visiting virtually every Local Government authority in Australia (except for Western Australia and the Northern Territory).

To say we knew Australia better than most Australians would have been an understatement. I can still recall the night life in the seaside towns of Glenelg in South Australia and magical Yeppoon on the Capricorn coast of Queensland. We also marvelled at the magic of sunrise in the Australian outback. Extraordinary memories of extraordinary places where Madeleine and I shared the most exciting and endearing times ever.

Life was great at home. The Springvale shopping centre was only 30 minutes away and was awash with exotic ingredients suitable for Mauritian cuisine.

Madeleine was in her elements having everything she needed within easy reach to cook the fantastic meals that everybody enjoyed. In 2001, we had another granddaugher Tyneisha, born in Canada to our son Michel and Canadian daughter in law Debbie. We enjoyed the company of our loved ones, especially the grandchildren.

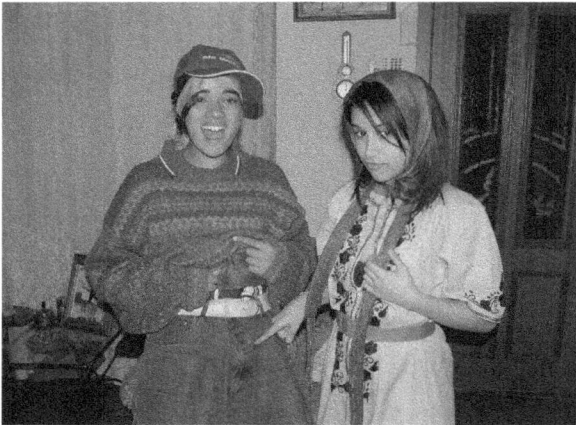

Jennifer and Annabelle imitating Gpa and Meme

In November 2006, during a visit to the doctor, Madeleine commented that she was suffering from pains in the right arm and also pointed out that she had not had a mammogram for quite a long time, some five years. She had the test a month later and we had a call from the doctor asking us to see him immediately. The mammogram had shown signs of possible breast cancer. We were in a state of shock.

We met with Dr Leigh Reeves, a breast cancer specialist surgeon in Berwick. He confirmed that Madeleine had breast cancer. In that instant, our whole world fell apart and Annabelle, our granddaughter literally hurled herself backwards and hit the wall with disbelief. I was numbed to find that breast cancer was with us and not something that others had. Madeleine herself was shocked and I could see tears running down her cheeks. I will never forget this moment. It was a reality check and suddenly we saw life in a completely different perspective. Immediately, priorities changed and only the things that mattered came to the fore, mainly love for each other and good health.

Madeleine had her last cigarette on Sunday January 28, 2007 before admission to hospital for breast cancer surgery. She never smoked another cigarette again.

The surgery took place on January 31, 2007 at St John of God Hospital in Berwick. A sentinel node in the right arm pit was excised using a gamma probe and found not to have any evidence of malignancy. The cancer lump itself in the right breast was excised but the 40 mm long tumour was found to be more extensive than had been apparent on the mammography scans. The surgeon cut through and removed the cancer cells and a specimen was sent for pathological examination.

The tumour was identified as invasive ductal carcinoma. The technology used to detect the spread of the disease was incredible. A radioactive dye was introduced into the cancer itself then by scanning the spread of radioactivity it was possible to map its extent. We were lucky that it was comparatively small and could be surgically removed. Furthermore, the breast cancer had not spread to the lymph nodes in the right arm pit.

Madeleine and I were very concerned by the seriousness of the situation and valued the incredible support from the family with some 15-20 family members turning up at the hospital to be with Madeleine before and after the operation. Madeleine had come through the operation well and we were all further relieved when Dr Leigh Reeves later confirmed that the surgery had been successful.

The local Breast Cancer Foundation provided support by giving Madeleine a hand stitched head rest, a custom made linen bag and other printed material to help her recover from the operation. This touch of kindness, at a time of great emotional upset and sadness, was deeply appreciated and welcomed by us both. The surgery was followed up with radiotherapy five days a week for five weeks. A further concern was that Madeleine had a pacemaker on her right side immediately above the right breast.

The pacemaker had been inserted on the right side of her chest under the skin, to remedy an irregular heartbeat (arrhythmia) some 10 years earlier. Care had to be taken to ensure that the radiotherapy did not affect or interfere with the pacemaker. I was taking no chances. Having alerted the pacemaker distributor, cardiologist, oncologist, radiotherapist and other parties to Madeleine's situation I initiated a teleconference between them to ensure appropriate steps were put in place to protect the pacemaker.

Follow up scans and tests after the radiotherapy revealed that the breast cancer was under control and contained. We rejoiced at the good news. However, I could not forget that Madeleine's mother Thérèse also suffered and died of a breast cancer that metastasized to other parts of her body. Whilst the breast cancer was beaten this time, I made it my mission in life to find and read anything I could on breast cancer and its causes. I discovered that a 73% survival rate of five years was possible. I prayed that Madeleine would be given another five years to see her grandchildren grow up and enjoy life with me. It was then that Madeleine and I met Dr Ian Haines who followed up the breast cancer surgery with hormonal treatment to minimize the risk of the breast cancer flaring up again. Little did we know that Dr Ian Haines was going to be our constant companion for the next four years.

Regular scans and further tests were also carried out under the supervision of Dr Maree Sexton at Frankston Private Oncology Centre.

It was during these radiotherapy sessions that we started to realize that there were a huge number of people who were suffering from cancer in one form or another. Cancer does not discriminate between young or old nor rich or poor.

Around the same time, Madeleine's cousin Cyrille was diagnosed with an invasive malignant brain tumour. He was given six months to live. This was a shock, as Cyrille was very close to us both, like a brother.

We used to spend time together on numerous occasions often dropping in to stay at each other's houses anytime we felt like it. He was the fittest in the family and if anyone would make it to 100 years old, that would have been Cyrille. When Madeleine was diagnosed with cancer as well, it was very difficult for us to break the news to him. He passed away almost exactly six months after his diagnosis. That was a very sad occasion for the family. In fact it was heartbreaking.

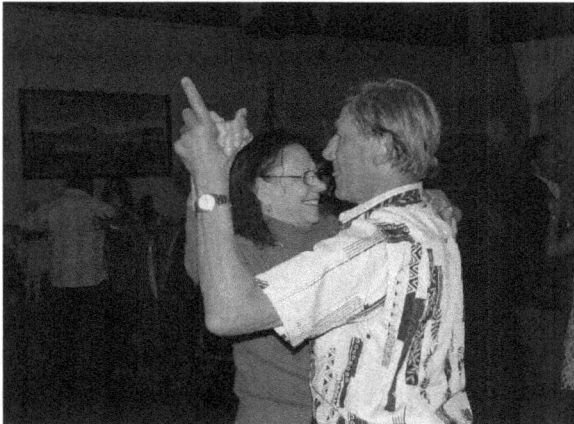

Madeleine dancing with Cyrille

Madeleine considered herself lucky in that the breast cancer was detected early. The pacemaker was replaced with a brand new one to avoid potential issues arising from the radiotherapy. The most challenging part was to provide support to Madeleine without overdoing it.

She was just incredible and totally trusted my judgement and assurance that things were under control. Madeleine kept a very positive attitude and prayed every night. Her faith in God was boundless. People visiting her could not believe how positive she was. Some people expected to see a half-dying corpse when they visited. Instead they saw a very vibrant person full of life and tremendously enjoying the company of her loved ones and true friends. Our eating habits underwent a radical re-think.

Fresh organic foods were on the menu along with sea foods, vegetables and other life sustaining foods. We ate meats only 2 or 3 days a week and avoided prepackaged or chemically treated products.

Suddenly it became very evident that Mauritian Cuisine was and still is as close as you can get to an anti-cancer diet. Mauritians have been using garlic, ginger, turmeric, thyme, mint, lentils, rice, onions, shallots, various greens, tomatoes, eggplant, tropical fruits, fresh seafood and a whole range of antioxidants within their daily diets for years. The use of garlic and ginger is a daily occurrence. As an example, the famous Mauritian Achar (vegetable pickle) must be very close to the best antioxidant combination that you could ever put together.

The research work done by Dr David Servan-Schreiber helped us enormously in regaining composure and moving forward. His book *'Anti Cancer - a new way of life'* became our bible.

This book is recommended reading for anyone affected by cancer. When David Servan-Schreiber, a medical scientist and doctor was diagnosed with brain cancer, his life changed. Confronting what medicine knew about the illness and the little-known workings of his body's natural cancer fighting capabilities, and marshalling his own will to live,

He found himself on a fifteen-year journey from disease and relapse into scientific exploration and finally, to health.

His is a moving story of a doctor's inner and outer search for balance.

Unfortunately, Dr David Sevan-Schreiber passed away on July 24, 2011. His work nevertheless remains a valuable contribution in winning the fight against cancer.

In summarizing his book, I can relate to Dr David Sevan-Schreiber findings through Madeleine's own situation:

- Traditional Western diet creates the conditions for disease;

- Sugar and stress feed cancer;

- The effects of helplessness and unhealed wounds affect our ability to restore health;

- The benefits of exercise, yoga, meditation and similar pursuits are undervalued;

- We should minimize environmental toxins in our homes; and

- We should consider a blend of traditional and alternative health care.

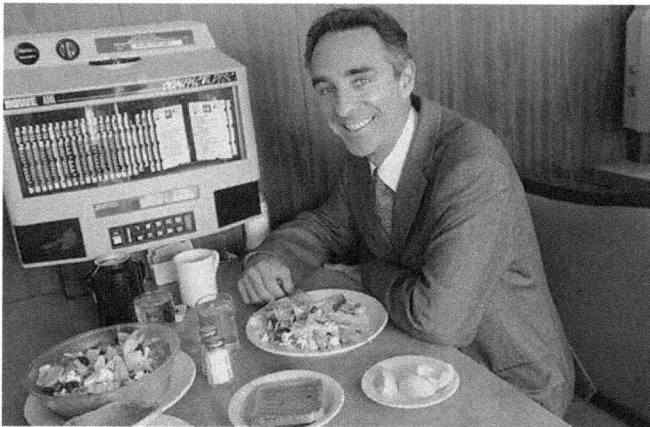

Dr David Servan-Schreiber

Meanwhile, I spent an enormous amount of time learning about breast cancer. So much so that one day, I was telling Madeleine about what I had read recently and about the progress made in its research; she responded in her own emphatic way by telling me that she appreciated my dedication in getting to know everything I could about breast cancer, but she wanted a break from discussions on the topic. I eased off and only brought up the subject when she did. However, she always told visitors how supportive I was to her and it was good to know that she truly appreciated my efforts. In the background, I was constantly searching for the results of new research in the battle to conquer cancer.

The task of looking after Madeleine was made very much lighter thanks to the incredible support from the whole family and especially Madeleine's brother Pierre and sister in law Lindy who undertook the daily grind of taking Madeleine to the radiotherapy sessions.

My employer the City of Greater Dandenong allowed me the freedom to be with Madeleine when she attended medical appointments. One of Madeleine's greatest pleasures in life was to enjoy the company of her grandchildren. Madeleine had always been a very non demanding person and put herself last on her own list of priorities. I was always number one on her list and she made sure that everything I wanted or needed was there.

It was exactly the same thing for me with her. She was my world. We had spent all our married life together and invariably did everything together. Losing her would kill me.

During one of the follow up sessions, the surgeon asked Madeleine whether she would consider plastic surgery to rebuild her right breast which had been partially removed. Madeleine replied: *"My right breast looks like a bull dog now; the only person who sees it is Clancy and he does not mind. I don't see any real reason to undergo plastic surgery."* That was Madeleine at her very best.

Madeleine's confidence and spirit were growing stronger. We were up and running again with the cancer experience left far behind us, apart from the regular checkups. Madeleine loved watching the travel TV series *'Getaway'* and always wished she had the opportunity to travel and visit the great cities of the world - Rome, London, Paris, Brussels and the like. The first Paruits (Madeleine's ancestors) who settled in Mauritius came from France and Belgium. The chance to visit the land of her ancestors was something I knew she would dearly love to do.

After cancer, your sense of priority changes and things that previously appeared very important become less so. My priorities in life had changed completely. You know the feeling that we all have: waiting for tomorrow to do things that we really ought to enjoy doing today. Well, my priority after the breast cancer scare was to make sure that Madeleine enjoyed life to the max and that we did things together that she would really enjoy. I had come to realise that caring for your loved ones and telling them you loved them was of the utmost importance. Tomorrow is not ours and could be too late to let others know how we feel.

I made the decision to take Madeleine on a world tour and visit the places that she had only seen on TV.

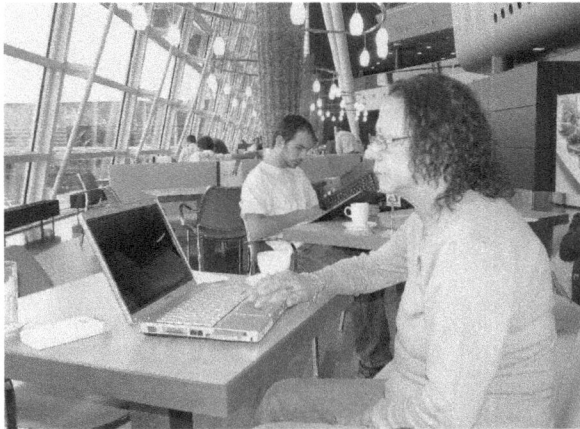

Madeleine tracking our itinerary

One night, I told her that I was making travel bookings for a seven week world tour for the two of us and that Annabelle and her boyfriend would stay at our place to look after the house and the dogs. The idea went down a treat.

Madeleine was over the moon and as we planned and organized the trip together I knew her dream to visit these faraway places was about to come true. She immediately started packing our bags for the world tour. She had incredible organising skills.

Chapter 5

Dream come true for Madeleine

**"One of my reasons for being alive is making one girl smile and making her happy for the rest of her life."
Anon**

We took off aboard Qantas flight no. QF 25 from Melbourne for Los Angeles on Monday August 13, 2007 at 10.55 am to arrive in Los Angeles on Monday August 13, 2007 at 10.45 am, earlier than we left Melbourne. Time difference gave us one extra day. I was watching Madeleine at Christchurch airport during the stopover and was so happy that at long last, she was realising her dream to travel around the world. The breast cancer scare had faded into the past and we were both enjoying our long deserved holiday.

Madeleine was really over the moon. She was in Los Angeles, the city where one of her favourite soap operas, 'Days of our Lives' was recorded. We only stayed 2 days in Los Angeles, but managed to pack in tour-guided visits to Hollywood Boulevard, Rodeo Drive, LA by night and a tour of Beverly Hills.

The traffic was absolutely horrendous. Even the taxi driver had difficulties fighting his way through it on our way to Wiltshire Boulevard. We were invited for lunch there by Marie Da Silva (auntie of Miguel – granddaughter Annabelle's boyfriend) who works for Ricki Lake, the popular US Ricki Lake Talk Show host. Marie was a wonderful host and a most engaging human being. We wished we could have spent more time with her. She has now dedicated herself full time to charity work for the Jacaranda Foundation in Malawi.

Marie could not stop telling us how impressed she was with Madeleine demonstrating such a positive attitude towards life despite the breast cancer experience. Madeleine and Marie bonded together in no time at all. They both had a very similar outlook on life, whereby nothing was too difficult if it meant helping or pleasing a fellow human being. Yet, neither of them would suffer fools gladly.

Only ten months earlier, breast cancer was putting our lives on hold. Cancer in the family, apart from directly impacting on the sick person, has a huge impact on all the loved ones.

The more you love that person the harder it gets. The evening and night walks in Los Angeles gave us those special moments that made our stay there more memorable. On Hollywood Boulevard, Madeleine marveled at the Walk of Fame where she could touch the imprints left by her favourite actors and singers. I can still see her comparing her handprint with that of Bette Midler.

I was very happy too, observing Madeleine 'all smiles' and enjoying life while we were in Los Angeles. The image of her sharing a smile with Shrek was so special it will stay with me forever.

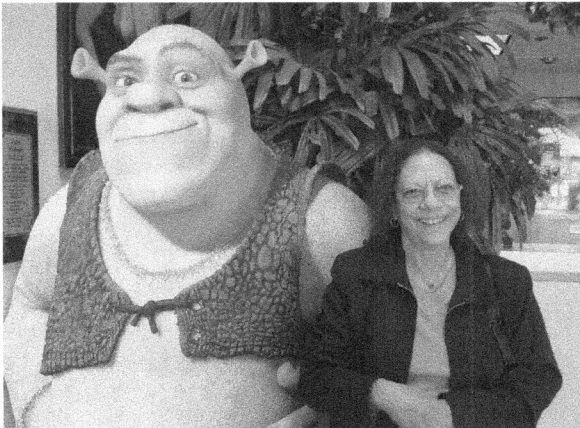

Madeleine with Shrek in LA

The trip through Beverly Hills gave us a peep into the homes of the rich and famous. Passing through Rodeo

Drive was another memorable experience with the designer clothing shops by Armani, Gucci and Coco Chanel, jewelers Cartier, Tiffany and Harry Winston, and exclusive couturiers where you needed an appointment just to get in the door. I can still see Madeleine admiring the lights of the forecourt to the LA Opera Complex, with ads promoting future Placido Domingo concerts. These moments will be cherished forever. I remember looking at her and considering myself to be a very lucky man to be part of her life.

We left Los Angeles on August 13, 2011 for Toronto, Canada where our younger son Michel had been living for a number of years. We were also looking forward to a first meeting with our beautiful granddaughter Tyneisha.

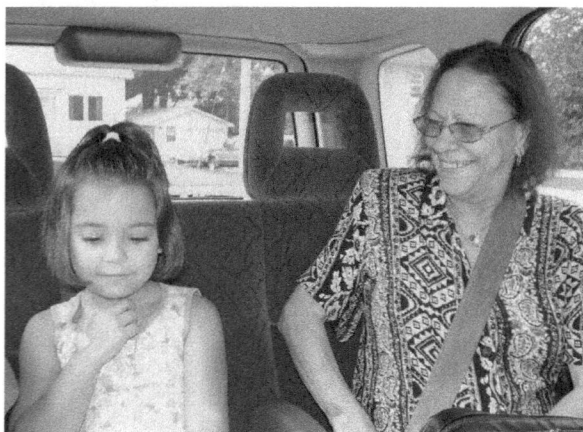

Madeleine with Tyneisha

We had a great reunion in Woodstock, some 100 km from Toronto, where Michel, his wife Debbie and the family lived. We were especially overjoyed to meet our granddaughter Tyneisha. We spent ten days there and it was just lovely getting to know the family.

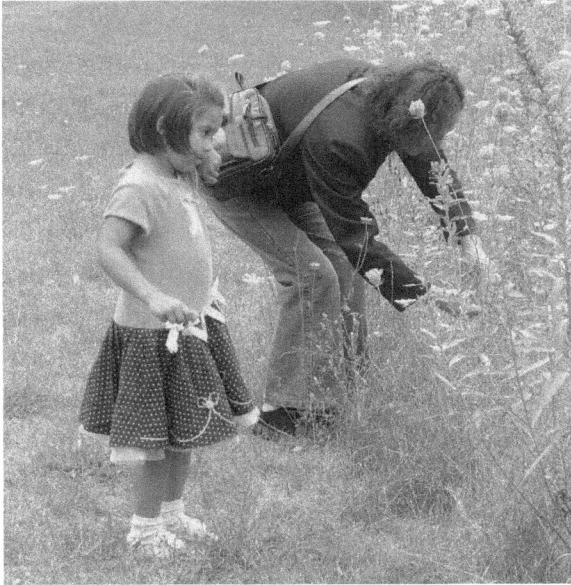

Madeleine picking flowers for Tyneisha

The sight of Madeleine walking with her granddaughter Tyneisha picking flowers by the riverside was a sight to behold. Tyneisha was very much like her sister Annabelle. Both have very sharp personalities with no hesitation to express their inner thoughts.

No doubt, these traits have been inherited from Madeleine. You are left in no doubt as to their opinion on things. Unfortunately, our stay in Woodstock was marred by the sad news that Madeleine's brother Guyto had passed away. This particular morning Madeleine had gone shopping with Michel.

I opened an email from a friend of mine in Mauritius, Gerard Cateaux, chief editor of the Week End Sunday newspaper. He was a good friend of Guyto's and they often played football together at the Racing Club. He had messaged to express his condolences to both Madeleine and myself. For some reason, the family in Australia had not been able to get in contact with us. It took some doing for me to pass on this bad news to Madeleine. Both she and Guyto were very close, sharing many things in common. Spiritually they could have been identical twins as they were very much alike.

He had been suffering from heart and lung problems for a while. Recalling our last time together prior to our departure from Melbourne, he repeatedly told Madeleine to enjoy herself and to make the best of her holidays. He was quite adamant on this point, almost as if he knew something was going to happen. I was also very sad about his death, as he was like a brother to me and we had great times together.

Knowing Guyto had recently experienced gratifying visions of the afterlife brought some consolation to Madeleine whose reaction had been to return home immediately. Guyto had been Madeleine's 'partner in mischief' and whilst it was hard to take in that he would no longer be there to continue the banter, inwardly Madeleine knew that he would always be with her in spirit. Our fond memories of Guyto will live on.

Annabelle represented us at the funeral. It was sad that we were not there to say goodbye but we were comforted knowing that by continuing to make the best of our holiday, we were in fact doing what Guyto had wished. We had already said our farewells in Melbourne without realizing. As already mentioned Guyto had been through two near-death experiences only months before and spoke about the *'bright lights and peacefulness he found on the other side.'* He also expressed the desire not to be brought back to life should he medically die for a third time. He said *'on the other side'* he felt really good and found spiritual tranquility and supreme peacefulness.

The long and entertaining discussions over drinks in the backyard patio at Michel and Debbie's home in Woodstock will live long in our memories. We visited Niagara Falls and that was an eye opener. No wonder it has become a worldwide attraction.

The entire Niagara Township revolves around the water fall. In town, a whole new entertainment centre has been created ranging from the casino to LA style attractions. We thoroughly enjoyed our visit there.

Madeleine's character and spirit endeared her to everyone. Debbie saw in Madeleine real inspiration from someone who really enjoyed life and always saw the good side of things. Madeleine's glass was always half full instead of half empty – albeit half full with scotch whisky which she enjoyed in the evenings before dinner. Debbie told us that our presence in their family made it a very special time for her. Before leaving Woodstock for Montreal, we were both very moved when Debbie burst into tears and told us she was really sad that we had to go our separate ways after spending ten lovely days together.

We arrived in Montreal on Monday August 21, 2001 and were received by Rowin from the Montreal Mauritian Community. He took us around the city, where we spent one wonderful day and night before catching our Swiss Airline flight LX 87 to Rome via Zurich. Madeleine's popularity from the *Recipes from Mauritius*' web site had caught up with her. Rowin told us that her recipes were well known and used throughout the whole Mauritian community in Montreal. Rowin was a real gentleman and before we left we invited him to come and visit us in Melbourne.

We landed in Rome on Wednesday August 22, 2007 at 2.00 pm. Madeleine had always been very religious and being in Rome was very meaningful to her. The very next day, we visited the Vatican and were most impressed with the very historic environment and the richness of the monuments and works of art. In fact, wherever we went, every corner of the place was steeped in Roman history.

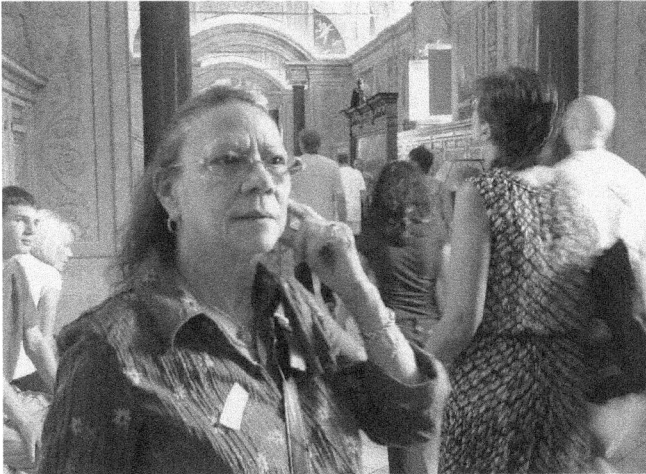

Madeleine in the Vatican, Rome

It was almost overwhelming. Seeing the Colosseum, the Vatican, the Dolce Vita precinct and the churches was reminiscent of the great city that Rome once was and to many, still is. We visited the Vatican Museum and the Sistine Chapel. The magnificence of the buildings and collection of works of art were beyond belief.

We also had a peep into the inside walls of the Pope's Vatican precinct. However, the Pope was not in residence, so we could not drop in for morning tea.

I observed Madeleine whilst we were inside the Vatican. She appeared very thoughtful, as if she had found some serenity and peace within herself. She was very quiet and only after we walked out of the complex did she start telling me how impressive it was.

The romantic enchantment of Rome was spellbinding as we dined 'al fresco' by the roadside and in pizzerias just like locals. We spent most of one afternoon wandering hand in hand as if through the laneways of history, exploring the squares and visiting the churches feeling like young lovers as portrayed in Federico Fellini's iconic movie 'La Dolce Vita'. Amidst the backdrop of these ancient yet spectacular Roman buildings and monuments, we shared some wonderful, magical moments together. *"I can still feel the presence of Madeleine walking beside me, holding my hand, as if it was only yesterday. These moments I will never forget."*

The only downside of our stay in Rome was losing my wallet at the Trevi Fountain, although Madeleine would have put an incident at the local restaurant above that. Again she took no shortcuts to let the proprietor know just how poor the customer service had been.

We left Rome on Friday August 24, 2007 from the Termini Station on the overnight Artesia Palitano sleeper train. We had a lovely dinner on board, befriended a very nice couple from the USA and were well looked after by Carlos, the compartment train attendant. Carlos also took care of the necessary passport stamping. It was a dream run: Madeleine and I travelling through Europe, sound asleep, with not a care in the world.

We arrived in Paris on Saturday August 25, 2007, having had a good night's sleep on the train. Settling in at Hotel Berkeley in Montparnasse, we were visited by Clarel Betsy and his friend Sharon. Madeleine knew Clarel well as a teenager and before he left for Paris to find fame and fortune. We spent some time in the hotel room talking about all sorts of things and reminiscing. We had lunch together before being taken on a fast but enjoyable sightseeing tour of Paris. Clarel knew every corner of Paris, despite the fact that he did not drive himself.

Poor Sharon worked very hard rallying us through the streets of Paris. We had a most incredible time seeing and experiencing in one day and night more than most tourists would see in a week. Mention any place and we would have been there. When we missed the way, we were taken through so many other places that we developed a very good feel for Paris.

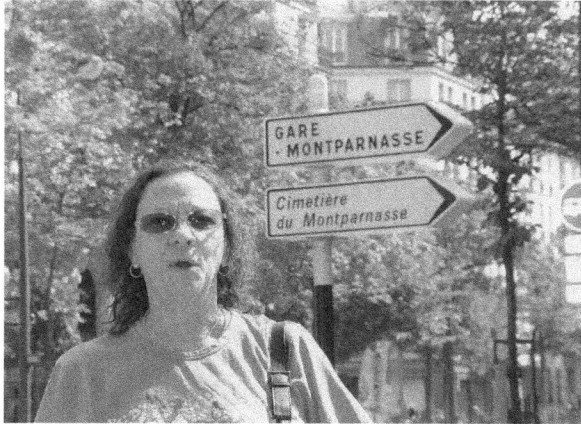

Madeleine at Montparnasse in Paris

Places like the Eiffel Tower, Arc de Triomphe, Place de l'Opera, Champ Elysees, Montmartre and many others, we knew them to the point of familiarity. Clarel kept us informed as to who lived where and what had happened in this place and that. He was very knowledgeable and could have made a fortune operating as a guide. His wittiness, complemented by Sharon's calmness and crowned by the direct talking of Madeleine made it a great day that we will never forget.

Clarel lost his wife to lung cancer and knew only too well what effect this terrible disease had on people. He was delighted that Madeleine had beaten breast cancer and was well on her way to a full recovery. Most of all, Clarel and Sharon admired the very positive attitude Madeleine had in the face of adversity. Her determination to keep enjoying life was very evident. As mentioned before, Madeleine was bursting with energy and I felt overwhelmed by her positive enjoyment of life and her ability to offer the hand of friendship to everyone she met.

Among the most memorable moments of our stay in Paris was dinner at a Mauritian restaurant, Tropic Beaugrenelle in Rue Beaugrenelle. Clarel, Sharon and two of Madeleine's fans joined us for this meal. Madeleine won the hearts of everybody dining there, especially when they learnt that she was the person behind the *'Recipes from Mauritius'* web site. The chef, owner of the restaurant and Madeleine finished the evening in the kitchen having a grand debate about Mauritian Cuisine.

We travelled to Lourdes from Gare Montparnasse in Paris. The first person to be miraculously cured in Lourdes was a Catherine Latapie in 1858 - coincidentally, the same family surname as Madeleine's mother Thérèse Latapie.

We both prayed and thanked God and the Virgin Mary for saving Madeleine from breast cancer. We also prayed for her future protection from this dreadful disease. It was very humbling to see people from all over the world, seeking the blessings of Sainte Bernadette.

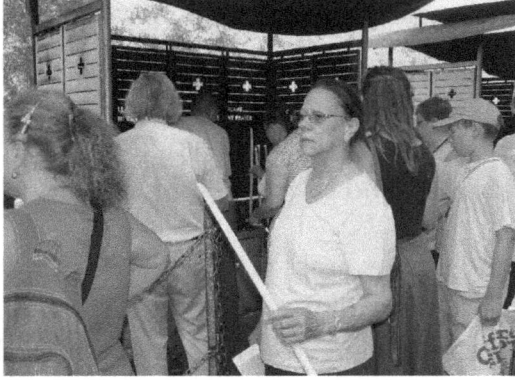

Madeleine lighting a candle in Lourdes

Madeleine lit a 50 cm candle a little way past the grotto where hundreds of candles had been lit by pilgrims. We then returned to the seating area where we prayed some more. We also visited the Basilique Souterraine de Pie X; a magnificent basilique built on top of the grotto where Bernadette saw the Virgin Mary. Masses were held continuously throughout the day and night for the almost continuous procession of pilgrims coming from all parts of the world. The atmosphere was so inspiring you could feel the intense devotion of visiting pilgrims. The happy memories of Madeleine and myself having breakfast on the 'terrasse' restaurant besides the Gave River, will remain another special moment that I will forever cherish. She was happy and truly living a 'dream come true'.

We left Lourdes the next day, with the promise that we would return. Our train journey on Tuesday August 28, 2007 took us to the small town of Orange, an old Roman settlement located very close to Mirabel aux Baronnies where the first Aliphon to settle in Ile de France (Mauritius) was born – 'Pierre Aliphon'. My grandfather Emile Aliphon was his 5th - making me a 7th generation descendant. Pierre was a 'tailleur de Pierre' or stonemason and was employed around 1780 by the Department de la Marine in France to work in the French colony of Ile de France (now Mauritius).

The train journey from Lourdes to Orange included multiple station stops throughout Provence and the Mediterranean coastline. Other than disembarking briefly in Toulouse and Arles, we could admire the landscape and the varying architecture, land use, hamlets and wide open spaces from the comfort of our railway carriage. The vineyards around Avignon were many and very reminiscent of our days in Mildura.

In Orange, we reported to Hotel Le Louvre to book ourselves in for the night. I overheard the 'concierge' talking to someone about a strong smell of ammonia in the hotel. We were shown to our room only to be blasted by fumes of ammonia coming from the bar fridge within the room itself which had obviously been leaking overnight.

With no other room available in the hotel and some sort of country convention in town meaning there were no vacancies available anywhere else, we had to open all windows and doors to air the room and sleep with the windows wide open. Had we been in the room the night before, we would not have survived to tell the tale. Someone from above was watching over us.

Orange itself was a town of contrasts, situated in Provence not far from the borders of Switzerland and Italy. Being one of the oldest Roman settlements in France it had a UNESCO listed Roman theatre backdrop and an Arc de Triomphe, both still in reasonably pristine condition.

The theatre combined scene and half circle seating with a huge arena and every year provided the setting for an annual opera show accommodating some 8,000 spectators. The year of our visit, they had 'Aida', with some of the best artists from France. Being a keen 'opera buff' Madeleine would have enjoyed watching 'Aida' in that environment.

The Arc de Triomphe in Orange had been erected by the Romans to commemorate their first victory over the Celts in France. Built by Julius Caesar in 49BC it was redecorated in 25 A.D by Tiberius. Dimensions: 90 m. wide, 18 m. high, 8 m. deep.

The triumphal arch of Orange had in fact three arches with rosettes, tympanum and nautical images to demonstrate Roman supremacy of the sea.

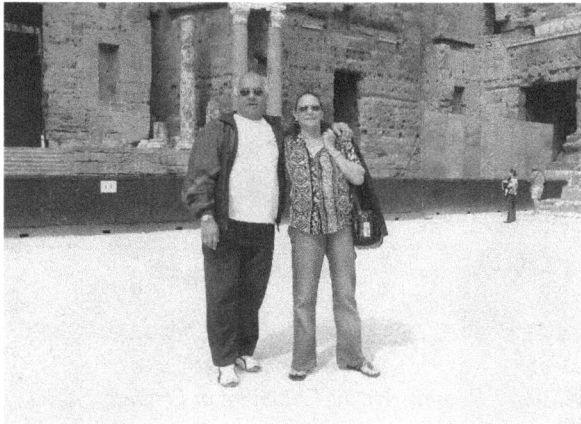

Madeleine and Clancy at Roman Theatre in Orange

The ornamentation was Greek, but the basic arch structure was Roman. Rocks were so perfectly cut that mortar was unnecessary. The Second Legion also built city baths, temples and the circus. The engineer in me was in awe of this structure.

Apart from the ammonia scare, Orange was just enjoyable and relaxing. We did a lot of walking and were pretty worn out.

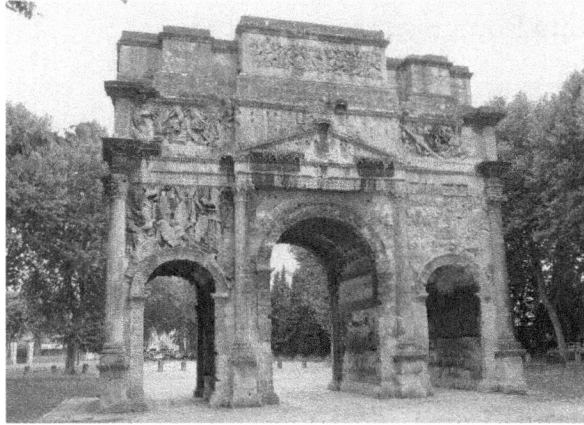

Roman Arc de Triomphe in Orange

Lunch in one of the rustic old Roman style buildings was another special moment to remember. We used Orange as a springboard for our visit to Mirabel aux Baronnies, Pierre Aliphon's birthplace. Remember, he was the guy who in the 1780's started the Aliphon dynasties in Ile de France (now Mauritius) and South Africa.

Well, I cannot begin to tell you how emotional I felt when Madeleine and I visited Mirabel aux Baronnies on August 29, 2007. The town itself was very small with a population of approximately 500 people and looked almost exactly as it might have been when first built. The architecture was very much in keeping with the Roman style and influence.

Within the main road intersection, the 250 years old Platane 'London Plane' tree, featured in old photos of the village square, was still there. As we stood under that tree it was as if we were reconnected across time – some 250 years ago, Pierre Aliphon must have stood under that very same tree. That's history for you.

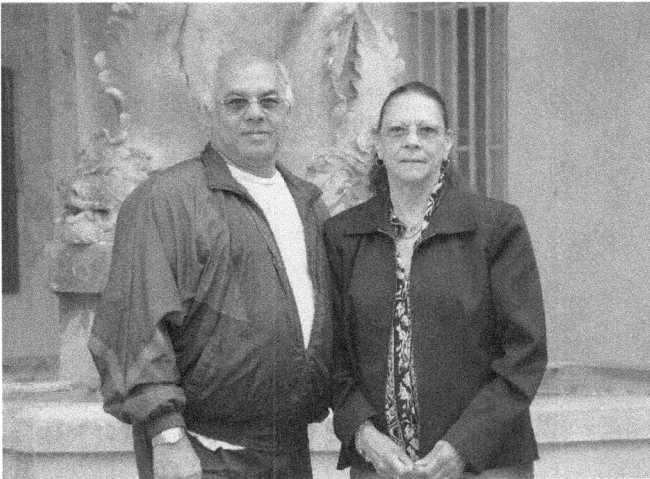

Madeleine and Clancy in Mirabel aux Baronnies

We wandered around the place soaking up the atmosphere. The public toilet within the Municipal Offices compound consisted of two long bricks on either side of a hole in the ground. To use the convenience, the visitor had to stand or squat on the bricks and complete their business. Madeleine went in and had to fold up her trousers just in case. She came out of the toilet with a big smile on her face, telling me about this ancient configuration.

The small Café des Amis within the village square did justice to its name. We were well received and after chit-chatting with the locals, we had lunch there. What a super friendly place. I was overcome by a very special feeling that part of me belonged to Mirabel aux Baronnies. A déjà vu experience you might say most probably brought on by my relationship to Pierre Aliphon and enhanced by the knowledge that his parents were most probably buried there. The time spent in Mirabel aux Baronnies had been a true reconnection in every sense of the word.

We left Orange for and stayed in Paris overnight, prior to travelling to the Champagne Ardennes district 130 kilometres east of Paris. On the train Madeleine kept herself very busy doing crosswords and reading. For as long as I had known her she had been doing crosswords on a daily basis. We were met by Yves Heeraman, a very learned and distinguished fellow who lived in Epernay. Madeleine's ancestors on the Paruit side came from the Champagne Ardennes district as did my father's mother's ancestors from the Bestel side.

Our visit to the area was a double reconnection with the past, stemming back to the late 1700's and early 1800's when Francois Bestel and Auguste Valentin Paruit left

France to find fame and fortune in Mauritius. Yves organized for the local paper to interview us as soon as we arrived and published an article about our visit the very next day. As a result of that interview, we established contact with a Paruit living in Reims.

Our visit to Reims included the famous Cathédrale Notre Dame de Reims and Le Palais du Tau. These two places were most impressive, filled with history and memorabilia of the past. Yves also took us to Epernay where he lived with his charming wife Hélène. There we visited the Maison de Champagne Mercier which included an incredible trip to the caves under Epernay where champagne was ageing for consumption by connoisseurs of good champagne.

I took a great photo of Madeleine standing besides the statue of Dom Pérignon in the forecourt of the Moet and Chandon establishment. We spent a delightful evening with Hélène and Yves, and shared a beautiful dinner together. Yves demonstrated his skills in 'sabrer le champagne', using the blunt edge of a sword to uncap the champagne bottle. Very impressive, so much so that on getting back to Melbourne, I ordered a sword to emulate him.

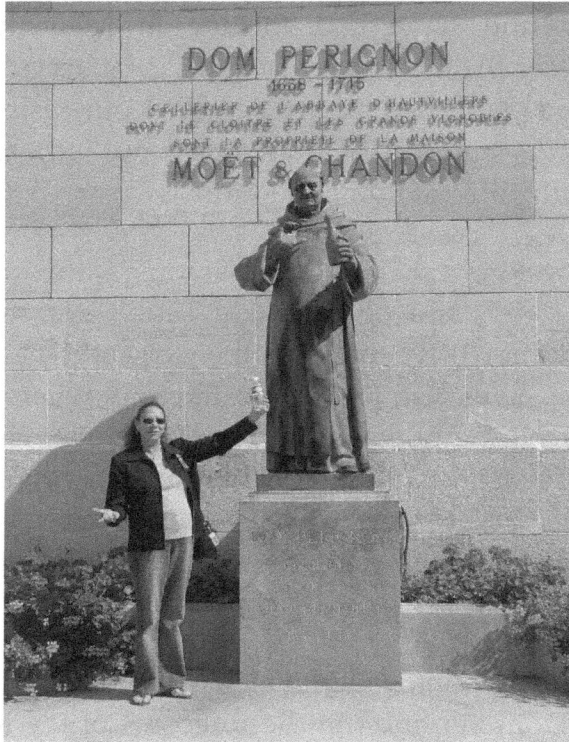

Madeleine with Dom Perignon in Epernay

Our next stop was Brussels where Madeleine's great great great grandfather was born although the Paruits were all originally from the Ardennes region not far from the city. For Madeleine, this was a pilgrimage to the birthplace of the Paruit who started the Paruit dynasty in Mauritius.

For us both the visit turned out to be something even more special.

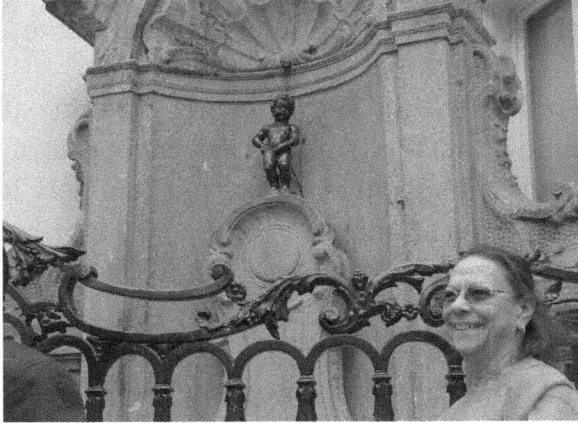

Madeleine at the Mannekin Pis in Brussels

Madeleine had always harboured the wish to visit Brussels and see the famous Mannekin Pis - a small bronze fountain sculpture depicting a naked little boy urinating into the fountain's basin. She had been given a Mannekin Pis key ring by someone who visited Brussels many years ago and I clearly remember her showing it to me just before we left for this world trip. The Mannekin Pis was symbolic of her desire to visit Brussels.

It was as if she was returning home. I had a similar feeling when we visited Mirabel aux Baronnies. We could both feel a special affinity with Brussels.

In fact, many Mauritians had migrated to Belgium, Brussels in particular. We also felt that of all the places we had visited during our world tour, Brussels would have been a real choice as a place where we could live.

We ambled through the city, enjoying the atmosphere and sharing some of the most memorable moments of our lives together. Our relationship had moved to a new level with our feelings for each other becoming stronger and deeper than anything we had experienced before.

We had reached the culmination of a true union between two people. Physically and emotionally entwined we were bonded as one entity in a way only 'death could make us part.'

Those memories will remain in my heart forever. This was my dream come true. The photo of Madeleine taken with the Manekin Pis was most symbolic as it represented that she had not only been there but it also represented the realisation of a lifelong desire.

We boarded the Eurostar on September 2, 2007 for Waterloo Station, London. The trip was thoroughly enjoyable and Madeleine was fascinated by the idea that she was travelling for part of the trip under the English Channel.

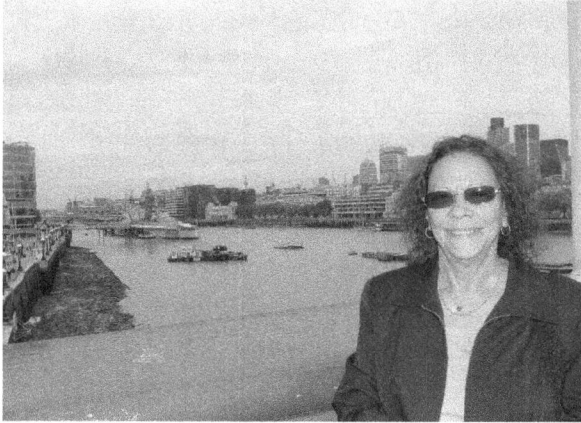

Madeleine in London

My mother's cousin Line and her daughters were waiting for us at Waterloo Station as we began a most pleasant ten days stay in London. We have known Line for a long time as my mother lived with her family after Line's mother died when she was still very young. Line also stayed at our place when she did her nursing apprenticeship at the Civil Hospital in Port Louis. Line has five daughters, three married and the other two living with her. Sadly she lost her lovely husband Willy to bowel cancer some time ago.

We were made to feel most welcome by the whole family including the sons in law, all of whom got on famously well with their mother in law. They were fascinated by Madeleine's very friendly 'what you see is what you get' disposition. They all just loved her and instantly accepted her as one of the family.

As I said before: *"Madeleine endears herself to everyone she meets."* Line's granddaughter Emily was a great fan of Madeleine's cuisine, and along with granddaughter Lara, found a special place in our hearts during the visit. In fact the whole Labiche Clan as I call them are living proof if ever proof be needed that love for each other is what makes life so special. I am very thankful that they got to meet Madeleine and establish a very special bond with her.

We visited the usual destinations in London. I also visited my mater alma City University in London, where I completed my Honours Degree in Civil Engineering. This brought back a lot of memories. Time flies. London has a special place in my heart. I spent some of the most enjoyable moments of my life as an undergraduate at the City University.

Madeleine and I were in Trafalgar Square where someone was feeding the pigeons, the usual tourist attraction and very popular for photos. Madeleine was given some corn seeds and the pigeons were flocking onto her. She emerged from under a cloud of pigeons to find a TV camera microphone poked in front of her.

It was a reporter asking why we were feeding the pigeons. We replied that it was the thing to do when in Trafalgar Square.

Little did we know that the local Westminster Council had just made the feeding of pigeons in Trafalgar Square a contravention.

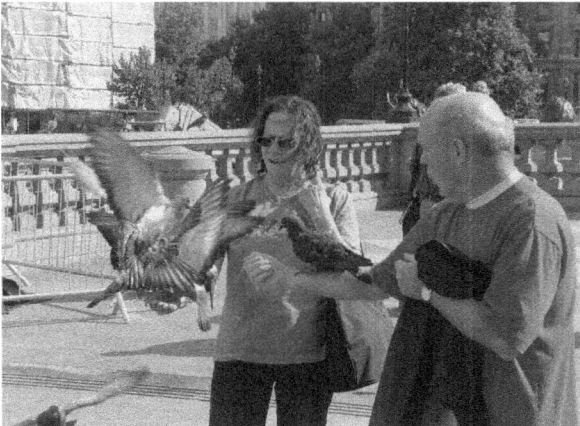

Madeleine in Trafalgar Square, London

This same afternoon, we appeared on British national TV talking about pigeons in Trafalgar Square. Line's daughter Arlette remarked: *"I was born here and lived here for some 30 years and never once appeared on national TV. You only spent 10 days in London and there you were, live on screen."*

We also visited the Tower of London much to Madeleine's delight. She was blooming with happiness and full of life. I have very many personal memories of the Tower of London where I had been on numerous occasions. Madeleine enjoyed the historical connections with the Royal family.

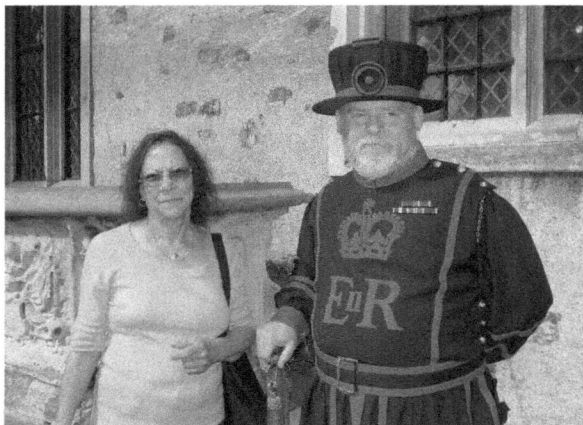

Madeleine with Tower of London 'Beefeater'

My grandfather Philippe married three times and his son Samuel, who is younger than me, lived in Bucknell, Oxfordshire - a small village not far from the university town of Oxford.

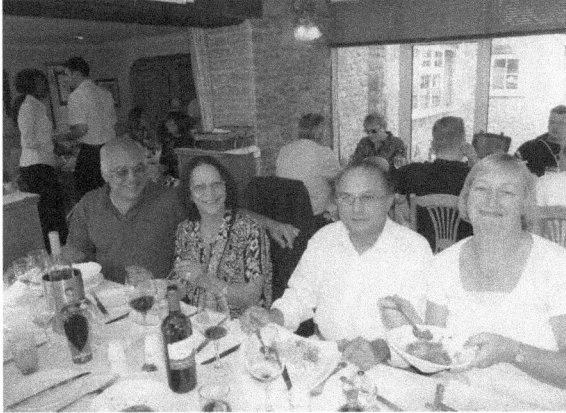

Clancy, Madeleine, Samuel and Anne

I had not seen Samuel since the 1960's when I left Mauritius for London to study. We spent three days there and it was very nice to catch up with him and the family after so long. Samuel just loved Madeleine's 'joie de vivre'. There too, Madeleine and I had special moments walking hand in hand down the lanes of Bucknell, admiring the medieval manor houses and stone cottages. Some of the buildings there dated back to the 19th Century. I can still remember the sight of the moss laden stonework and trees.

We also met with Madeleine's cousin Gerard Bechet in Bentley, not far from Edmonton where we stayed with Line, Maryline and MaryAnn.

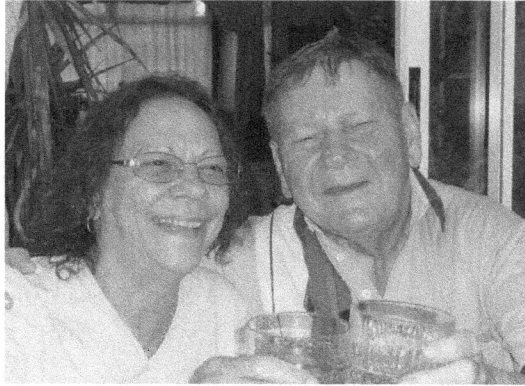

Madeleine with cousin Gerard

Gerard and family were very happy to see us and Gerard was especially delighted to see that Madeleine had fully recovered from her breast cancer operation. Gerard's mum who was Madeleine's auntie also died of cancer - yet another stark reminder of the family's encounter with this killer disease.

Our visit to the Bechet family coincided with Gerard's wedding anniversary. We were invited to stay on and celebrate. That night Gerard and Madeleine did celebrate with more drinks than Gerard could cope with. Madeleine as usual was still going strong. Just like Johnnie Walker. I have never seen Madeleine drunk – merrier and more lovable, but never drunk.

On Wednesday September 12, we took off from Heathrow Airport on Swiss Air flight LX 327 for Johannesburg, South Africa. We arrived in Johannesburg on Thursday September 13, at 9.10 am, to be met by my cousin Guito Aliphon's daughter Amanda. We stayed at Amanda's apartment for two days before flying to Harare, Zimbabwe to stay with Guito and his wife Mottie for ten days. Bringing photographic equipment into the country could have been a problem as it was illegal to take photos of public places or public buildings. However we passed through customs without any issues and with me keeping a very low profile as we did.

Harare was very barren both environmentally and people wise. The political situation and bad economic times had left all shops virtually empty. Only the select few could afford to buy imported food items and people had to queue for essential items such as milk and bread. We had ten really enjoyable days in Harare where we were made to feel most welcome. It was wonderful reconnecting with my cousin Guito and his family, and with his Dad who was the only surviving member of my mother's side of the family. Guito and Madeleine truly appreciated their evening 'Johnnies' - that is their evening Johnnie Walker Scotch whisky. Madeleine again stole the show, winning the hearts of each and every person she met.

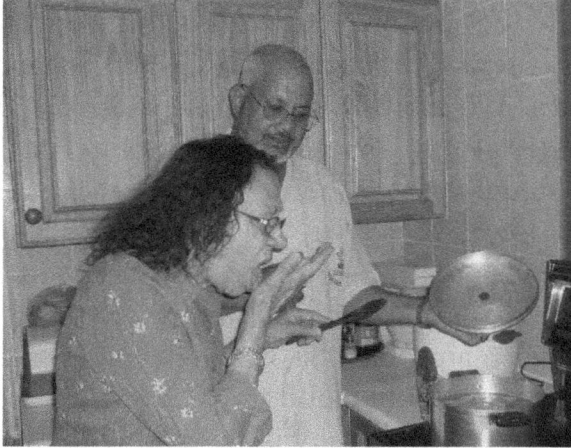

Madeleine tasting Guito's cooking

Yet again, her 'what you see is what you get' approach and her enjoyment of life on a day to day basis were greatly admired by the whole family. Sadly, all good things come to an end and we had to make our way back to Johannesburg, before boarding Qantas flight QF 64 for Sydney on Sunday September 23, 2007.

Whilst it was enjoyable to visit faraway places and family, it was good to be home again. We stayed for one week with our sister in law Wallis, who had lost her husband Guyto whilst we were in Woodstock. It was very sad to be in Sydney, with Madeleine's brother Guyto no longer around.

We were back in beautiful Australia to carry on with our daily lives and enjoy the company of the children and grandchildren, as well as the family and numerous friends. It was also time to organise the appointments for the periodic medical checkups to ensure that the breast cancer was well under control. It was September 2007, spring time and Madeleine was itching to get back to her garden with me pottering away by her side.

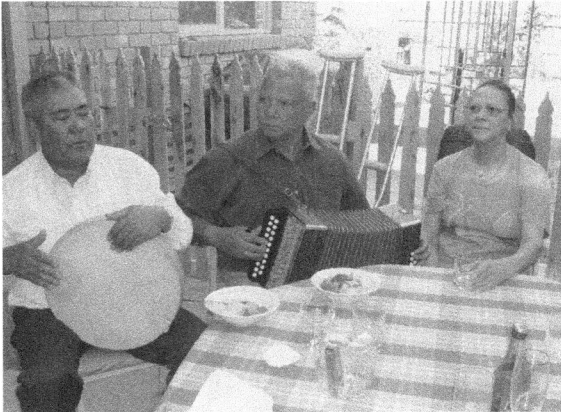

Madeleine entertaining Rodriguan friends at home

Living the dream had brought us closer than we had ever been before and we were both looking forward to spending quality time together not only in the garden but also by immersing ourselves in all the other projects we had on the to-do list now we were back home. Life had never felt so good!

Chapter 6

Cancer makes a comeback

"My cancer scare changed my life. I'm grateful for every new, healthy day I have. It has helped me prioritize my life." Olivia Newton-John

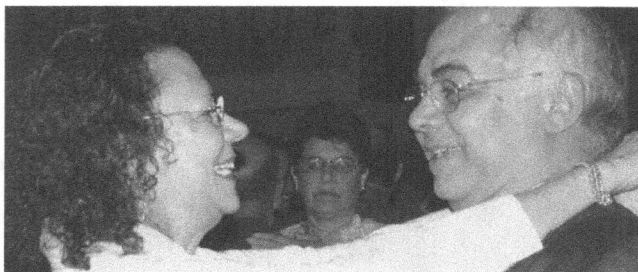

Madeleine and Clancy happy

We celebrated Christmas 2007 and the New Year in great style with the family around. It was very comforting to enjoy the company of the loved ones. We also enjoyed the many social events organised by the Mauritian community in Melbourne. Everything was hunky dory and life could not be better. The regular checkups for the breast cancer confirmed that the breast cancer was very much under control. Madeleine went back to her kitchen and prepared her delicious meals for all to enjoy.

The recipes for these dishes were also broadcasted worldwide through the very popular *'Recipes from Mauritius'* web site at *http://ile-maurice.tripod.com*

The breast cancer surgeon again offered Madeleine the option of undergoing plastic surgery for her right breast. She declined by repeating that I was the only one to see her breast and that I did not mind, even if it did look like a bull dog. We were really happy, enjoying time with each other and the company of our loved ones. Breast cancer was well behind us. The year 2008 sped past very quickly and all the monitoring confirmed that Madeleine had well and truly beaten the disease. Madeleine was as radiant as ever and enjoying life again. I had never seen her so happy.

In early November 2008, Madeleine suffered from minor bleeding and her GP referred her for an abdominal CT scan, to be followed by further tests. I had to ring around to find a gynaecologist who would give us a follow up appointment. Fortunately, on Tuesday November 11, 2008 there was a gap in Dr Maurice Litchter's appointment calendar and I rang Madeleine from the office letting her know that I was on my way to pick her up for the appointment. We were stunned when Dr Maurice Litchter confirmed that Madeleine had what appeared to be malignant ovarian cancer.

It was traumatic to say the least. He sympathetically updated us on the situation and organised for us to see one of the top ovarian cancer surgeons in Melbourne, Associate Professor Thomas Jobling. Up until that moment we may have felt a bit seasoned but nothing could have softened the impact of this terribly bad news. Madeleine and I had just recovered from breast cancer and we were getting our lives back together again. We were both dazed by the news and again the only thing I could think of was *"We had to beat this one too."*

The children and grandchildren were shocked at the news. The only thing to look forward to was that both Madeleine and I were to attend the André Rieu Melbourne Concert in Melbourne that Saturday. This was to be our last great outing together.

I felt very sad for Madeleine, who despite the bad news, kept her coolness and trusted me implicitly to guide her into action. As usual, her determination and fighting spirit were there poised for whatever it took to battle on. I don't know whether she cried in my absence (she probably did), but I cried on and off when not in her presence, fearing the worst case scenarios. However, we somehow both put on a brave face when we were together. We met with Associate Professor Thomas Jobling at his Brighton surgery.

He confirmed the diagnostic and organised for Madeleine to be admitted for surgery at Epworth Freemasons Hospital in East Melbourne on November 19, 2008.

As usual, I spent the whole time with Madeleine whilst the loved ones came in and out during the day to offer their support. She was very courageous and did not show any signs of nervousness or negativity at all. Externally, she put on a very brave and happy face. But inwardly, I asked myself the question *"Would she be as worried as I was?"*

I felt sure she would have been, but somehow she trusted me implicitly and put on a very positive front.

We had an exceptional ovarian cancer surgeon standing by in one of the best world class hospitals that you could have access to. The rest was up to God, the surgeon and Madeleine herself.

Madeleine even found courage to dance in her bedroom with the surgery gown on, whilst waiting to be picked up and wheeled into the operating theatre. *"I can still see her dancing in her favourite red 'ballerina' shoes that we bought in London."* That's the sort of person she was. *"We had always believed that between the two of us nothing was impossible, not even this latest challenge which life had chosen to thrown at us."*

Together we were more resolute than ever to overcome whatever lay ahead. Madeleine's toughness prevailed as usual.

Madeleine went into surgery around 7.00 pm and the operation took some three hours, during which I was pacing up and down the waiting room. Dianne, our older son Gerard's partner, kept me company and made sure that I did not freak out. She provided me with great support when I needed it most. Thank you Dianne.

I had a phone call at 10.30 pm from the surgeon, Associate Professor Thomas Jobling, who advised that the surgery went well.

He found a high grade carcinoma size 65 mm on Madeleine right ovary, with a smaller sized high grade carcinoma on Madeleine's left ovary, metastatic carcinoma in two other spots within the abdominal cavity. Madeleine's ovaries and uterus were debulked and the metastatic carcinomas cleaned up. The cancer was diagnosed Staged IIIC Ovarian Cancer. Stage IIIC is the final Stage III classification. The next level of ovarian cancer is Stage IV, which is no longer curable. The five-year survival rate for patients with Stage IIIC ovarian cancer is 31.5 percent. I was determined that Madeleine would be within the 31.5 percent.

The surgeon also told me something that I kept to myself for years and only very recently told some people about it. He said to me: *"The cancer will come back."* At that precise moment I made the decision: *"I will personally take care of this challenge in due course"* and lived with those words reverberating in my head for years. I was never going to tell Madeleine that, nor any of the children and grandchildren at the time. I kept that promise to myself and did not tell anyone about it until after Madeleine passed away.

Madeleine came out of surgery reasonably stable, but her lungs played up and she was placed in intensive care with constant monitoring for some five days. Her breathing had to be assisted, but her courageous approach helped to overcome this setback.

When Brandon, our grandson saw her with all the tubes and drips, he got very upset, but his Meme Madeleine told him that there was nothing to worry about.

At one point, Madeleine's condition was hovering between bad and very bad and I started having serious concerns about her condition. She however, promised me that she would be OK. True to her word, she picked up again and was transferred to her hospital ward bedroom.

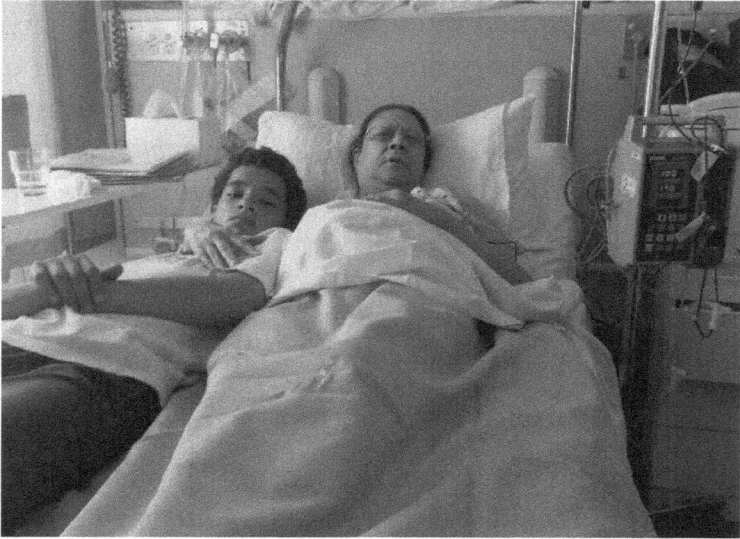

Grandson Joshua with his Meme Madeleine

There she won over the hearts of the surgeon, doctors and medical staff with her more than positive attitude. I took time off work and stayed with her every day, only going home to shower, sleep and look after the dogs.

One night, she felt that someone was caressing her legs. Little did she know that staff had fitted one of those massaging devices to her legs to promote blood circulation. We both had a good laugh about that the next day.

Madeleine received the best of care at Epworth Freemasons' hospital and we were indebted to all their medical staff for the total dedication shown not only to her but to all the patients.

Family, loved ones and friends visited Madeleine in hospital and offered support for her quick recovery. Everybody was astounded by her positive approach in her second encounter with cancer. Fans of her Mauritian Cuisine website *'Recipes from Mauritius'* sent get well messages on a daily basis and I updated Madeleine on the support for her coming from worldwide. When strangers from all over the world tell you that they are praying for you and wishing you well, you cannot help but feel spiritually enriched. These acts of genuine caring proved to be a real tonic in Madeleine's recovery.

Talking about prayers, Madeleine prayed regularly before falling asleep and that gave her a lot of courage, confidence and determination to carry on. In particular, she prayed to Saint Mary MacKillop, a 19th-century nun who became Australia's first saint in October 2010.

Whilst I do not pray regularly myself, I found myself praying when the going got tough. At home, she lit a candle to Saint Mary MacKillop every night. I have kept this going ever since.

Madeleine left hospital on November 27, 2008 and we were looking forward to spending Christmas 2008 and the New Year with our loved ones.

I was determined to make sure that she had everything she needed to make her comfortable and to ease her back to full health. My Louloune (Madeleine's nickname) was back home and I was the happiest man on earth. We renewed acquaintance with Dr Ian Haines, oncologist at Cabrini to discuss the way forward. We were already seeing him periodically for the breast cancer follow up and once more we would be relying on his expertise to guide us through the next challenge. Ian also advised us that the cure rate was less than 50%. I was not sure that Madeleine quite registered that at the time. As usual, she would always look at me and whatever I recommended, she would go along with. Madeleine commenced chemotherapy at Cabrini on December 18, 2008.

Ian was treating her with a combination of drugs specifically designed to interfere with the growth of cancer cells and to ultimately destroy them. Carboplatin was an alkylating agent whilst Paclitaxel (Taxol) belonged to the group of antineoplastics medicines. However, we were told that the growth of normal body cells could also be compromised and that there were often unwanted side effects.

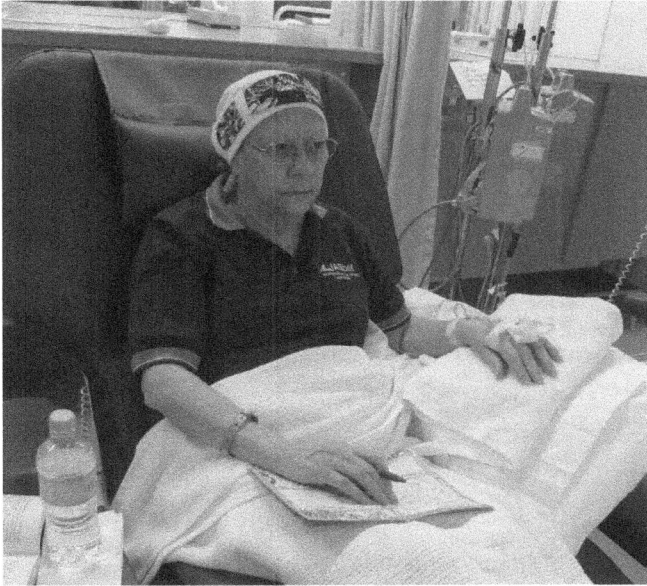

Madeleine at Cabrini undergoing chemotheraphy

I received a number of emails from well-meaning people suggesting that Madeleine's cancer should be treated with natural products instead of the conventional treatments.

We chose proven conventional treatments supplemented with a healthy organic choice of foods. It is interesting to note that Taxol was, in a way, a type of natural product, as it was originally derived from the bark of the Pacific Yew tree (Taxus brevifolia) by botanist Arthur Barclay in 1962, and later discovered to have the cytotoxic properties capable of destroying cancer cells.

Madeleine, who was normally very prone to allergic reactions, immediately felt the side effects. With ruthless determination she had made up her mind that she would just have to learn to live with them. As well as having the occasional nose bleed and little mouth ulcers, she had tingling fingers and her taste buds went funny.

She also suffered from abdominal pain as a result of the hysterectomy operation. Fortunately, the side effects gradually diminished over time. On top of everything, she was feeling fatigued but thanks to her fighting spirit she did not let any of that get in the way of her chemotherapy treatment. She was a true champion and was more than intent on winning this second battle with cancer. Once more Madeleine's strength of character endeared her to all the staff and nurses at the Cabrini Oncology Daycare Clinic.

The chemotherapy was initially planned for weekly sessions over a six months period, with regular blood tests prior to treatment to ensure that Madeleine's immune system was standing up to the onslaught. Ian also organised for tumour marker CA-125 & CA-15-3 tests to monitor and measure progress. CA 125 is mainly used to monitor the treatment of ovarian cancer. The CA 15-3 marker is used to monitor the response to treatment of breast cancer and to watch for recurrence of the disease.

A decreasing level generally indicates that chemotherapy has been effective, while an increasing level indicates tumour recurrence.

Meanwhile, I researched all I could about ovarian cancer and around the same time, started researching about the occurrence of breast and ovarian cancer in the family.

Of the 200,000 women who are diagnosed with the cancer worldwide, ovarian cancer is the fifth leading cancer claiming the lives of over 100,000 women per year. Consequently, the prognosis associated with ovarian cancer is not very good. As I mentioned before, the five-year survival rate for patients with Stage IIIC ovarian cancer is 31.5 percent. I was constantly haunted by Associate Professor Jobling's words: "the cancer will come back" and despite keeping this information away from Madeleine I was still determined to make sure she would be within the 31.5%.

What would you do in these circumstances? Well, I opted for the positive approach and prayed that the chemotherapy would control the cancer. The loved ones did the same oblivious to the knowledge I had gleaned whilst researching the causes of and prognosis for ovarian cancer.

The weekly trek to the Cabrini Oncology Daycare somehow brought hope to what could only be described as a desperate situation. I for one was not going to let go and painstakingly explored every avenue possible to beat this dreadful disease.

It was particularly distressing to learn that most ovarian cancer cases were not caught early as was the case for Madeleine. Things did not look good.

It was obvious from my research that one of the reasons why ovarian cancer went undetected was because the symptoms associated with it were minor, and often women were not concerned enough to want to go to the doctor. Diagnosed early, the prognosis and survival rate for these situations were known to be as high as 98 percent. Secondly, there were no real screening tests yet available to pick up this type of cancer. Often, doctors didn't know for sure that ovarian cancer was present until they could see it on an ultrasound or detect cancer cells from tissues extracted in a biopsy. Regular medical checkups and early detection were crucial. To promote this message, Madeleine and I co-founded the *Madeleine Philippe Cancer Foundation (Aus) Inc* to promote and create awareness of the need for the early detection of both breast and ovarian cancers.

No symptom or pain in the breast or abdominal area should be left unchecked, especially if breast or ovarian cancer is known to be present in the family.

It was an eye opener to see so many cancer patients attending the Cabrini Oncology Daycare. They came from every section of the community, young and old, rich and poor, famous and ordinary people.

The doctors and nursing staff offered hope to all. Their caring and patience were limitless and nothing was too difficult or unimportant.

Madeleine and I saw in them an immense source of support and encouragement. It was almost like an insurance policy that would keep the cancer under control. Over and above, they offered hope, love and understanding. One common element with all the patients was that their priorities in life underwent a complete and radical change, whereby the importance of family, love for each other and tolerance prevailed.

Sadly there were many lonely patients who did not have the support of loved ones and no one at home with whom to share their joys, pain and grief. To see such solitude at a time of great need was truly heart breaking. One of the most painful moments was to see young adults coming for treatment.

I was particularly affected by a young girl of the same age as our granddaughter Annabelle undergoing chemotherapy. Madeleine attended the Cabrini Oncology Daycare every Tuesday, with the help of her brother Pierre and sister in law Lindy.

They picked her up from home, dropped her at the Cabrini Daycare Clinic and stayed with her until I made my way there directly from work and took over for the rest of the day. Thank you Pierre and Lindy, we are eternally grateful for your love and assistance during those difficult times. I will never forget that. A very sharp contrast from some who just did not love or bother enough to care.

When Pierre and Lindy could not make it, Madeleine's brother Jean stood in and took Madeleine for her treatment. On June 9, 2009 our oncologist Ian congratulated Madeleine on being such a good patient. He named her his "Star AAA+++" patient as she had responded so well to the chemotherapy. Madeleine had two more chemotherapy sessions and was subsequently given the all clear. She was in remission.

We were so happy that it was like being in love again for the first time. Once more, we were looking forward to enjoying life again without cancer hanging over us.

Madeleine was happy with a permanent smile on her face and bursting with energy.

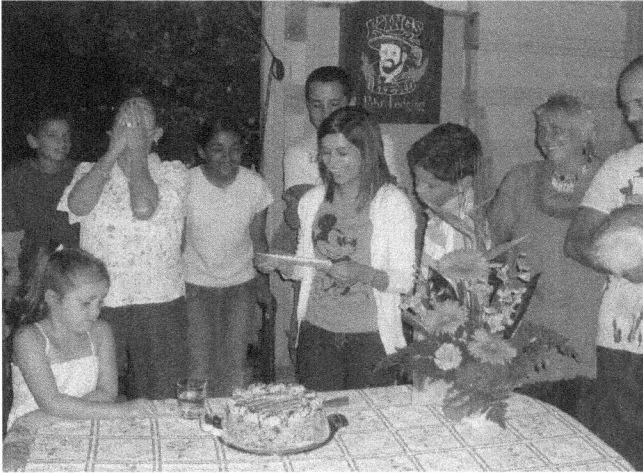

Madeleine's birthday celebrations

The whole family was happy, the children and grand children especially rejoiced that their Meme was safe. Madeleine and I started going out again to some community events.

The six months of chemotherapy had somewhat affected her immune system and we had to be careful not to expose ourselves to the unnecessary risk of infection, such as colds and flu. We were also planning to travel again and our first trip was to visit the family in Mauritius. Our priorities had changed radically with the important things becoming so obvious. We had started to see life through very different eyes. After surviving this life threatening situation, our main concern was to spend as much quality time as possible with our nearest and dearest and to focus on helping others in need.

Telling those closest to us how much they were loved and appreciated became second nature. Material pleasures became non events and little things that previously would upset us did not matter anymore.

We were living day by day and enjoying every precious minute. We stopped living for a tomorrow that might never come. Past events were left behind, apart for the happy memories that were locked in for future reminiscence.

As a result of our experience with cancer, we noticed the changing attitude shown by people we knew. In truth it was in many ways a painful reality check to see how friends and acquaintances could be classified in a very definitive manner as to *'those who really cared'* and *'those who did not'*.

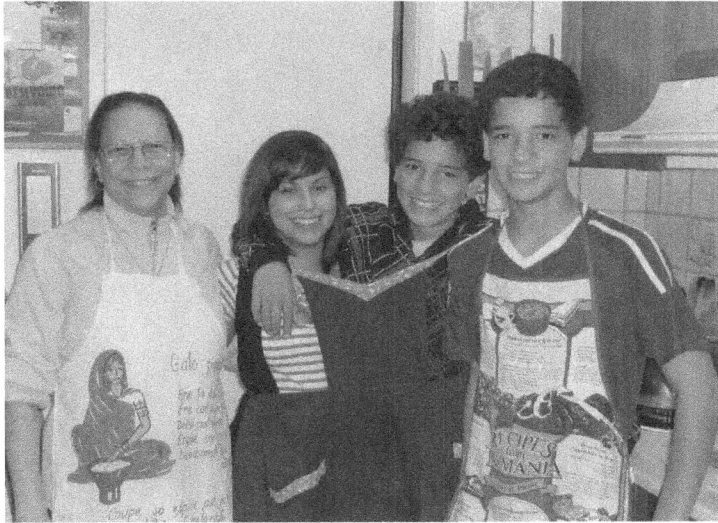

Madeleine with grandchildren Annabelle, Brandon and Joshua

All too clearly we found out who our real friends were. I always said to our granddaughter Annabelle *"If you could count on one hand five real friends, you would be a very lucky person."*

I also remember my mother Daisy saying: *"Grandchildren always gave you unconditional love."* I can say that this is very true.

Madeleine was back into the kitchen we had renovated with state of the art cook top and new bench tops.

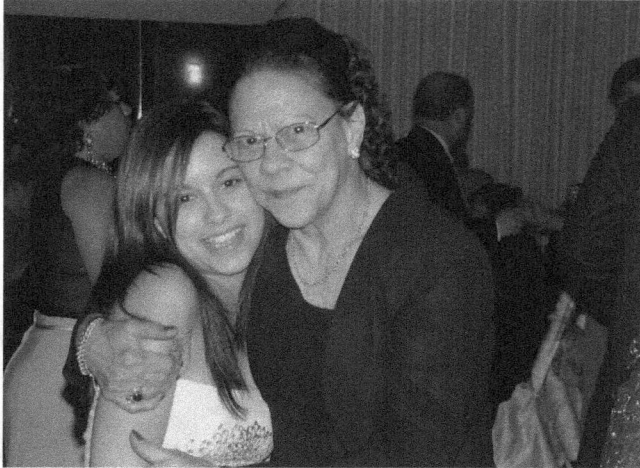

Madeleine with Annabelle at a community event

Leave Madeleine in the kitchen and she was in heaven! We were all enjoying her culinary skills and we were planning new recipes for the web site, including a series of DVD's that would promote Mauritian Cuisine even further. Despite her illness, Madeleine was determined to continue expanding and sharing her passion for cooking with others worldwide.

Everybody who met Madeleine was absolutely astounded by her positive spirit and 'joie de vivre'. That was my beautiful Louloune (Madeleine) in full stride again. I was very happy too!

We also were going out more often and participating in community gatherings.

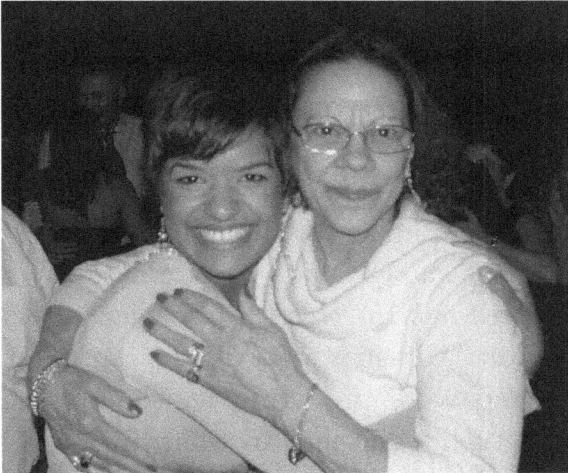

Madeleine with the young lady from Rome

One very unforgettable moment occurred one evening when Madeleine and I were at a dance in the Springvale town hall. A young lady walked over to Madeleine, gave her a big hug and started crying. When Madeleine asked her why she was crying the young lady explained: *"I live in Rome all by myself and at times I can get really homesick. When I do, I go to your website, get the recipe for one of my favourite Mauritian dishes and cook it. The aroma and taste of the food make me feel like being at home again and I am no longer home sick."* By then Madeleine was crying too. A very special moment indeed which made all our promotional work feel so worthwhile.

On October 6, 2009, we met with the very distinguished Dr Pravin T P Kaumaya from Pittsburg University. He was visiting Melbourne, Canberra, Brisbane Gold Coast and Couvan Cove to give lectures and attend a symposium on cancer research. He had accepted an invitation to be a patron for the *Madeleine Philippe Cancer Foundation (Aus) Inc*. He said: *"As a Mauritian expatriate, I would be honored to be involved in your foundation."* He had also met with Ministry of Health representatives in Mauritius, who were preparing legislation to introduce clinical trials of his vaccines in Mauritius. He also said: *"Breast Cancer is a major problem in Mauritius. So let us all put our various expertise to help our compatriots."* He was also a fan of Madeleine's *'Recipes from the Mauritius'* web site. In an email prior to the Melbourne visit, he asked me: *"Is Madeleine the lady who has the Mauritian recipes on the web?"*

Living in America he loved the site. He went on to say: *"I have used these recipes to create many dishes especially the briyani (mari bon). Please thank her for bringing these recipes to us."* Madeleine's reputation in Mauritian Cuisine knew no frontiers.

Madeleine had her regular monitoring tests for cancer activity. Everything had been going according to plan until Madeleine started suffering the odd aches and pains, with some breathing difficulties.

There was some concern in relation to cancer activity on one of her lower vertebrae. However this turned out to be a false alarm.

Meanwhile, an examination of the family history led to the discovery that there was an alarmingly high incidence of ovarian and breast cancer in the family. Madeleine's great grandmother, her mother, two aunties, sister and cousin all died of either breast or ovarian cancer. Madeleine's sister died of secondary ovarian cancer at 44 years of age. I had read about the Jack Brockhoff Foundation Familial Cancer Centre which offered genetic tests for such families. Under a government program run by the Peter MacCallum Cancer Centre in Melbourne, Madeleine undertook the DNA tests in November 2009 to find out if she carried either the BRCA1 or BRCA2 gene fault. The tests would take 6 months to complete with the results available in April 2010.

At the start of February 2010 Madeleine was aware of a persistent numbness in her left leg and was having lower abdominal pains. To make matters worse, the tumour marker tests indicated an increase in levels leading to Madeleine resuming chemotherapy treatment (paclitaxel & carboplatin) on February 18, 2010. Madeleine's tummy had also started swelling with a build up of fluid (ascites) caused by the secondary ovarian cancer.

The ascites had to be extracted by means of a needle inserted into the pelvic area in what had to be the most daunting and unpleasant procedure to date.

Two litres of turbid orange fluid were drained from her tummy and tests later confirmed the presence of metastatic high grade carcinoma, this time originating from the ovarian rather than the breast cancer.

To this day I still carry the image of Madeleine as she bravely endured this ordeal. Not once did she complain or hesitate to undergo this, or indeed any other treatment that was required. She would look at me and if I nodded, she would just go along 'no questions asked'. She still had total faith in my judgement and that of our consultant, Ian.

As the treatment proceeded, Madeleine suffered more and more from miscellaneous symptoms associated with the cancer, the medication she was taking and the complications arising from her illness. She was eating very little at this stage and as she could not taste her food properly it made her reluctant to eat anything at all. She had tingling feelings in her limbs and in the abdomen. The numbness in her left leg became so bad that for the most part she had no feeling in it at all. The hernia suffered during the original ovarian surgery along with the presence of secondary cancer made matters worse.

The normal constipation that she already had from the chemotherapy became more acute. Bowel movements became very difficult. Cancer was back with a real vengeance.

On March 4, 2010, during the chemotherapy session she had acute chest tightness and the palms of her hands became bright red. The carboplatin component of the chemotherapy had to be stopped. Ian cancelled the next weekly session and allowed Madeleine to rest for one week before resuming treatment. On the same day, a semi permanent device called a PICC was inserted into Madeleine's upper arm as the medical staff had been experiencing some difficulty finding a vein through which to administer the chemotherapy treatment. This would remove the need for the insertion of injection needles at future sessions.

On March 18, 2010, the treatment side effects and the abdominal pains still persisted. Madeleine's overall condition was not improving and she had started losing weight which was not a good sign. Despite all these problems, Madeleine kept a brave face and carried on with the battle. One evening after returning from treatment, I looked at her and tears were rolling down my face. She looked me straight in the eye and said: *"Don't cry in front of me as you will make me cry too."* Since then, neither of us cried in front of each other.

On April 19, 2010, the result of the DNA tests taken in November 2009 came back. It confirmed that Madeleine was a carrier of the BRCA1 gene fault.

This finding explained why she had developed breast and ovarian cancers. Mutations in this gene are responsible for approximately 40% of inherited breast cancers and more than 80% of inherited breast and ovarian cancers. This result also meant that this genetic test would be made available to family members over the age of 18 to determine whether or not they had inherited the same gene change.

On May 23, 2010, Madeleine had erratic fever and was admitted to Cabrini Emergency Unit. Thankfully, the fever subsided and she was allowed to return home. Her temperature, weight and fluid intake were closely monitored and she had started taking pain killers to ease the aches and pains. Despite all the ups and downs and continuing weight loss, Madeleine persevered with the chemotherapy.

Things appeared to be improving and on July 1, 2010, the day before my birthday, the CT scan and the tumour markers did not indicate any sign of cancer whatsoever. I remember saying to Odile Ternel, a close relative of ours that this was the best birthday present ever. A miracle had happened and Madeleine had beaten cancer again.

I told everybody the good news and we were all very happy. Madeleine also said to me how much was looking forward to being in remission again.

For some strange reason, I said to her that we would wait for the results of the follow up tumour marker tests just to be doubly sure.

We were driving to hospital for the next treatment, and we were both looking forward to Ian telling us that Madeleine had beaten cancer once again. Madeleine was so full of expectation that Ian would confirm that she was indeed in remission.

That was not to be. The tumour marker test results indicated a flare up of secondary ovarian cancer, with very high levels of cancer activity. I can still see the disappointment and despair on Madeleine's face and in her eyes, looking at me and seeking an explanation. I did not know what to say and was totally speechless. Even the nurse who was looking after Madeleine was shocked.

We were now in August 2010. Obviously, Madeleine's body had stopped responding to the paclitaxel and carboplatin chemotherapy. Cancer activity was increasing and on September 23, 2010, she was having her 60th treatment. By then, the pain was so intense that Ian started prescribing the strong pain killers Endone and Oxycontin, in addition to sleeping pills. The fluid buildup in Madeleine's abdomen had started again and on September 28, 2010, some 2.2 litres of ascites were drained from her abdominal cavity.

On September 30, 2010, the chemotherapy treatment was changed to a gemcitabine/carboplatin combination. I recall the nurse reading that the situation was getting desperate, wishing Madeleine all the very best hoping that this new chemotherapy combination would work.

I also remember sneaking into Ian's surgery without letting Madeleine know, and bluntly asking *"Ian, what are the chances of Madeleine getting cured?"* He looked at me, then said: *"30% or less."* Madeleine was in trouble and there was nothing that I or anyone else could do. I kept this assessment to myself.

Madeleine accepted the situation heroically. She did not say anything and was somehow lost in her own thoughts.

We both knew what each of us was thinking. We did not have to exchange any words - our eyes did the talking and it was not looking good. As promised, we retained our tears for each other's sake.

On returning home, we both put on a bold front. Madeleine said to me: *"I think that I am not getting out of this one this time."* I responded by saying: *"We are not beaten yet. Only God knows."*

I also remember saying: *"Even if there is only one chance in a million, we will be going for it."*

The whole family, friends and loved ones were astounded by the bad news. No one could believe that after this long grueling battle with cancer which Madeleine had won three times, she was not going to make it the fourth time.

On reflection, I believe this was the turning point in Madeleine's five year battle with cancer. Madeleine's body had taken a battering and was showing signs of weariness. Madeleine's own fighting spirit was dimmed and not long after, fatigue set in and I could feel that she was giving up the fight. She also said to me: *"I have been praying so hard, but my prayers are not being answered. No one is listening!"* I responded by saying: *"Praying is good for you."*

My faith in God was seriously challenged and I was asking myself some serious questions, with no answers forthcoming. I just could not believe that Madeleine despite her loving nature, belief in the Almighty God and all the good that she did, had to suffer like this. There was no justice!

"Why should someone like Madeleine who was so caring, beautiful, loving, full of life, with so much going for her, have to go through this ordeal and torment?"

Chapter 7

Madeleine's Waterloo

"There are times when a battle decides everything, and there are times when the most insignificant thing can decide the outcome of a battle." Napoleon Bonaparte

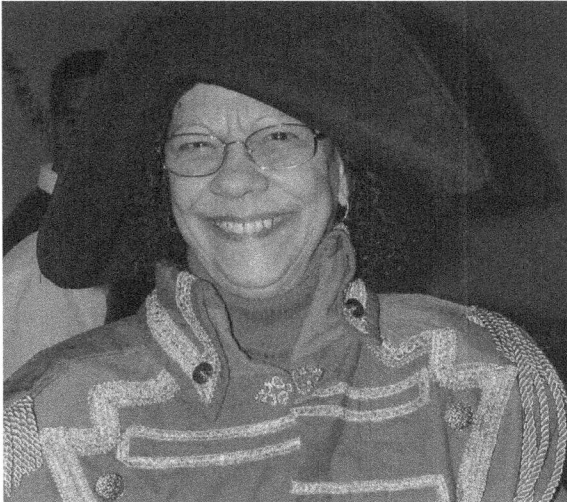

Madeleine in battle mode

Why Waterloo? The first Paruit d'Esmerys, Auguste and Henry (Madeleine's direct ancestor) came to Mauritius in the 1810's and both fought as young soldiers (17 & 16 years old) in the Battle of Waterloo, which Napoleon Bonaparte lost to the Duke of Wellington in Belgium.

During the first two weeks in October 2010, Madeleine had to be admitted four times at Cabrini Hospital either as an emergency patient or to drain her abdomen from ascites build up. Some 4.5 litres of malignant yellowish fluid were extracted. On two occasions, she was admitted with fever and released on the same day. Despite all this, she underwent a second session of chemotherapy with the new drug combination of carboplatin and gemcitabin. Her courage was exemplary. Her weight by then had reduced to 62 kilos. Due to her weakening condition, the chemotherapy sessions were stopped and on October 29, and November 8, 2010, 2.2 and 3.8 litres of malignant ascites were drained from her abdomen.

Things were not looking good at all. On October 27, 2010, she was diagnosed with an enlarged heart with left ventricular failure and a mild degree of pulmonary vascular congestion. CT scans on November 1 and 4, 2010 revealed significant coronary artery disease (cardiac failure) and metastatic nodules, particularly dense around the lower pelvis. I was losing my soul mate, the love of my life, my friend and my companion of 34 years. Our loved ones, family and friends rallied around Madeleine and me.

However, I felt helpless and kept a brave front for Madeleine. In her presence, I smiled, expressed hope and encouragement to battle on. In private moments and very often whilst driving alone or travelling to and from work, tears would stream down my face. Madeleine too, felt that she was losing the battle. In my presence, she held on and never gave up nor showed signs of despair . She kept smiling but her eyes told me a different story. She was worried about me being tired, having to wake up three to four times every night to care for her, afraid that she was going and leaving me to care for myself.

I re-organised home to make all conveniences available within reach of her bedside, including bedside stick to assist her in getting out of bed, walking frame, her drinks, puzzles and crosswords, emergency telephone setup, television remote controls, books and the little things that made life easier and more comfortable for her. Whilst she could still get out of bed, albeit with some effort, I continued to go to work but came home for lunch every day to make sure that she was alright. As things deteriorated, my employer, the City of Greater Dandenong kindly granted me permission to work from home.

She was admitted to Cabrini hospital on November 8, 2010 with fever and other complications and was discharged on

November 12, 2010 after she told Ian that she wanted to go home.

CT scans indicated digestive malignancy, malignant neoplasm of retroperitoneum and peritoneum, as well as malignant secondary ovarian cancers. She had more chemotherapy sessions on November 18 and 25, 2010 which she struggled to cope with.

On November 29, 2010, she had a further 5 litres of malignant ascites drained from her abdomen. Jean, one the nurses at 'Imaging Cabrini' became particularly fond of Madeleine and took great care of her, making sure that she was well looked after. You just knew that she was really moved by Madeleine's courage and willingness to fight on. Jean, you are a real credit to your profession, very compassionate and caring; your empathy and understanding provided great comfort and support at a time when we needed it most.

The relationship between Ian and Madeleine became a very personal one. They teased each other whenever the opportunity arose. Madeleine was getting very weak and had to be taken to Ian's surgery in a wheel chair. He told Madeleine to rest for the incoming week and he would reassess her condition the week after. Madeleine responded: *"If I am still alive the week after!"* to which Ian replied: *"If you are not alive next week, please don't come and see me!"*

At this point in time, Ian spoke about Madeleine being admitted to hospice care. I said: *"No!"*

I totally refused and said that as long as I could look after her, she would stay home. Madeleine was worried about my work situation and I said to her: *"Don't worry, I have great support from the Council. If things get bad, I will retire and look after you full time."* I was told later that she had spoken to a few loved ones and said: *"I am worried about Boum (my nickname) and I don't know what would happen to him if I die."* She was more worried about me than herself. She was told not to worry and that they would look after me.

Increasingly, Madeleine needed assistance with even the simplest of tasks. I had to help her shower herself and do the little personal things. She even needed help to stand up. Madeleine and I developed impromptu routines that made life easier for her. In order to get up and move around, she would either use the walker with someone in attendance or I would bend over to her and she would grab my neck and me her waist. We would then synchronize our movements and she would rise to her feet. I would then walk backwards with her following me, just as if we were dancing together.

Sometimes she would say to me: *"I am getting stronger. I can get up easily."* The truth was we were becoming more synchronized in our moves but I would smile and agree: *"Yes, your legs are getting stronger."* We were having our last dance routines together.

We were also having the visit of palliative care nurses whose help was greatly appreciated as indeed was the overwhelming support given by the whole family. Around this time, our elder son Gerard and his son Brandon moved to our place virtually full time to assist both Madeleine and myself. Annabelle our granddaughter came and cleaned up the bathrooms. Pierre (Madeleine's brother) and his wife Lindy, as well as Doreen, our ex daughter in law, stayed at home to look after Madeleine when I had to go out. Gerard's girlfriend Dianne also dropped in to assist in more ways than one. Other family members and close friends popped in and out to boost morale and offered to prepare meals for us. The loved ones were closing in on Madeleine to give her as much support as they could. I will always be eternally grateful for that.

Even our Maltese Shih Tzu 'Baby' would regularly appear in our bedroom just before bedtime and sleep on the side of the bed where Madeleine slept. She would stay there until we put her in her own basket.

I remember Madeleine saying: *"Why are you doing this, am I going to die."* To this day, I believe 'Baby' knew that things were not going too well and in her own special way was doing her best to protect Madeleine from what lay ahead.

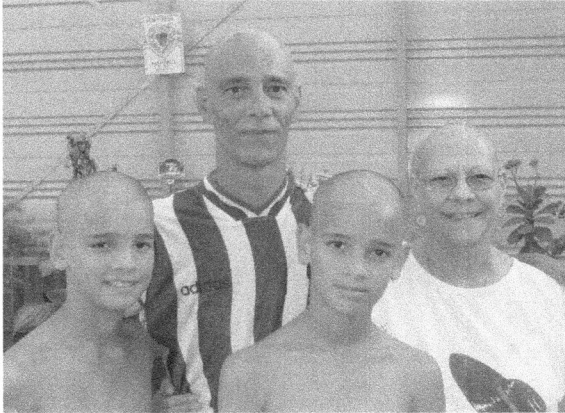

Gerard, Brandon and Joshua shaving their heads in solidarity with Madeleine

Madeleine's condition was declining fast. One day, Gerard was helping her up the steps from the patio into the house when she fell down on her knee. Psychologically this seemed to affect her as she became reluctant to leave her chair. Our dancing move and grasp was the only way she felt confident in moving around safely, apart from when she used the walker. She demonstrated an incredible resilience in taking things as they came. However, the loss of taste and her inability to eat spicy foods or have an occasional drink affected her badly. She said to us: *"There is no point me being in the kitchen as I cannot prepare or eat my favourite dishes."* This was a full body blow to her; she was no longer able to spend time doing what she enjoyed best - cooking.

She had also lost her passion for crosswords and puzzles, she could not even have the odd whisky and her praying became intermittent.

The weakening in Madeleine's condition seemed to magnify our ability to cope. Somehow a renewed spirit came up from within giving us the will and determination to continue the fight. Madeleine herself displayed so much courage in the face of adversity. She never gave up despite the fact she was totally dependent on others. Every now and again, she would say to me: *"It's about time that you get to know where things are in the house."*

I played dumb and pretended not to understand, but she knew how I felt. She would also ask me to spend more time with her, like coming to bed early. I really treasured those moments. When the pain was not too bad, we would cuddle each other into a display of affection. We sort of knew that the days were numbered.

During December 2010, Madeleine had four more chemotherapy sessions, 4.5 and 5.0 litres of malignant ascites were drained from her abdomen. The nurses at the Centre continued to display considerable compassion and support always ensuring Madeleine was made as comfortable as possible. Despite further complications with erratic temperature, aches and pain, Madeleine kept smiling. I kept smiling too.

I took leave from work during most of December 2010 to be with and look after her full time. That was the least that I could do. She would have done the same for me.

Christmas 2010 was to be the last big family occasion together with all Madeleine's loved ones gathered around her. She struggled to make it to the lounge room, but insisted on distributing the Christmas presents to us all. She was very febrile and I can still see her doing her best to be cheerful and loving to everybody. Only three days earlier, she had 5 litres of malignant ascites drained from her abdomen.

Madeleine needed round the clock care. I was monitoring her medication (including painkillers), weight, temperature, blood pressure, blood sugar level and liquid intake constantly. She had lost a considerable amount of weight. The fluid in her abdomen was increasing all the time and had now migrated to the left leg which had to be kept permanently in an elevated position. Gerard and I took it in turns to massage the leg in order to push the fluid back into the abdominal cavity. Anti swelling socks had to be worn to contain the swelling and to limit the fluid migration. It was utterly heartbreaking to see Madeleine suffering in this way, especially as there was nothing more we could do. As she could not get up easily, she had to take fluid through the use of a baby cup fitted with a straw.

She took all in her stride and rather than complain she invariably managed to smile and kept her joyful approach to life by regularly making jokes about her condition. Incredibly, she was still battling through with courage and hope, when there was really none forthcoming. I remember her teasing Dianne after the latter spent all afternoon cleaning up the mess she left in the bathroom and bedroom. Thank you Dianne. I will never forget what you did for your 'Mamma'.

I would be up three or four times each night to bring Madeleine to the bathroom or to attend to her needs. Sometimes, in her sleep, she would almost wake up and talk to her deceased brother Guyto or her mother Thérèse. This occurred several times and each time I almost felt their presence in our bedroom. Sometimes, in the morning she would ask: *"I don't know what is happening, I cannot help but think about my brother Guyto."* You may remember from earlier chapters, Madeleine and Guyto were very close and had a very special relationship as sister and brother.

On December 30, 2010, she underwent another chemotherapy session. The subject of palliative care was brought up again to which I responded that I would keep her at home for as long as I could. Finding herself alone in palliative care would be enough to kill her, just through sheer grief. That would kill me too.

We needed each other's presence badly and there was nothing that would separate us. Like they say: *"Till death us do part."* She knew that and so did I.

We battled on for the New Year and celebrated as best we could. On January 2, 2011, Madeleine was in so much pain and feeling so tired that we had to take her to emergency where she was admitted straightaway. The next day, things improved slightly. However, in the early hours of the following morning I received a call from the ward nurse: *"Your wife is crying and saying she's scared. She is asking for you, could you please come."* I was by her bedside at 5.00 am to comfort her. She fell asleep straightaway.

On January 4, 2011, Madeleine had 3.0 litres of malignant fluid drained from her abdomen. The swelling in her left leg had reached her foot and was getting worse. Some fluid migration had spread to other parts of her lower body and was now affecting the right leg.

The scans and other tests confirmed a worsening of the digestive malignancy, secondary malignant neoplasm of retroperitoneum and peritoneum, as well as malignant neoplasm of ovary and adenocarcinoma metastatic. I had a long private discussion with Ian who advised that Madeleine had not long to go. She was dying. I was losing my soul mate, wife, confidante and companion of 34 years. She was my everything and I was totally dedicated to her. She was my reason for living. I was devastated. My whole world had totally collapsed.

But I had to keep going and display a brave face for Madeleine. Ian also issued instructions for Madeleine to be transferred into a private room and provided with the utmost comfort possible.

Despite all this, Madeleine kept her calm and even asked to be taken in a wheel chair to the hospital courtyard. Gerard, Michel and I took her down one afternoon. One carrying the oxygen bottle, the other pushing the wheel chair and me making sure that everything was going OK. We sat down in the canteen and she had a small piece of cake and a sip of coffee. She truly enjoyed that break from the hospital room. She was constantly making jokes and keeping us entertained.

We stayed with her all the time, day and night, helping with her daily routines and keeping an eye on her. Little things became very meaningful for her, like being next to the window and admiring the blue sky scenery.

At that point in time, I advised all her loved ones, family and friends that Madeleine did not have very long to go. She gradually became more febrile, but showed extreme courage in all this despite the odds. I also told her fans worldwide that we were losing her.

Gerard and I took turns staying with her overnight to make sure that she had the presence and continued affection of her loved ones. We also knew what to do to assist her with her little problems and to make her comfortable. Either Annabelle, Jennifer or Dianne also stayed to keep her company.

During these night time vigils she would frequently hold some sort of conversation with either her brother Guyto or her mother Thérèse. We would wake up, look at each other and feel the very strong presence of the departed loved ones. We were totally convinced that through her talking, these deceased persons were there. On one occasion, she was in bed completely helpless and hardly able to move.

That did not stop her from sitting up, bringing her arms forward and saying *"Maman"*, as if reaching for her mother Thérèse. I felt strangely relieved that both her mother and brother Guyto were there for her.

The days and nights we spent with her were our final 'Au Revoir'. In between her sleepy moments, she regained consciousness and uttered a few words to us. On one occasion, her suffering was so intense that I could not help but ask the doctor: *"How long is this going to be?"*

I could not bear to see her suffering that much. At one point she reached for me and said: *"Aide moi."* (Help me), and as I sat there I realized for once there was absolutely nothing that I, or indeed anyone else could do.

Those two words *"Aide moi."* (Help me) broke my heart beyond repair. The only words of comfort I could muster were: *"Ian is doing the best he can."* In the past, I had always been able to find a solution to any problem she had. This time, I was totally and utterly helpless. This was the most heartbreaking moment of my life.

Whilst I was sitting in the bedroom, watching my loved one slowly fade away, I wrote this to two of my close colleagues at work:

"I am currently in Madeleine's hospital room watching her slowly fade away. She has lost the will to fight and is slipping away fast. The doctor has advised that it is only a matter of time. Am just devastated to find that such a lovely and caring human being has been almost totally consumed by this dreadful disease. She is now on morphine to ease the pain.

Don't know what more to say. Will keep you posted and give you a call when things settle down. Am seeing the doctor tomorrow re path from here. Clancy"

I also wrote to her fans worldwide:

"Am sad to announce that Madeleine is losing her 5 year battle with breast and ovarian cancers. She has been admitted to Cabrini Hospital in Malvern (Melbourne) with terminal cancer."

Responses poured in by the hundreds from worldwide:

"Dearest Clancy,
I am deeply saddened by this and pray that God will give her strength. Thinking of you both constantly.
Sending love from all."

"Hi Clancy

What can I say, my friend...I can't even stand the thought of being in your shoes and I pray I never have to! I also pray for you and your lady and may God be by your side. I know the pain is too great for you to have any positive thoughts and it is only human for you to be angry and bitter however you should also consider yourself lucky!... Lucky that you are one of only a few people who have met their soul mate in this lifetime and have felt the love and devotion that comes with such a special relationship! Think of the special times you have shared and of the lady who stood strong by your side and lit up your life with her smile, her laugh, her spark and all those qualities that make up MADELEINE!

My thoughts are with you both and I am only a phone call away if you need to talk...I can even come to the hospital."

Madeleine's loved ones came to visit every day - the children, the grandchildren, other family members and close friends.

My brother Josian who was very close to Madeleine, came to be with us almost every evening. Madeleine's brothers and sisters in law travelled from their holiday camp in Anglesea every other day and offered support. Madeleine's brother Jean could not hold back his tears. He knew that his sister did not have long to go.

I could not have managed to hold things together during Madeleine's final days if it had not been for the love and comfort of those nearest and dearest being there for us. Father Richard Rosse, a friend of the family also saw Madeleine, prayed with her and administered the 'Last Sacrament'.

On the night of February 10, 2011, Annabelle and I were spending the night with her. She was labouring to breathe, but otherwise comfortable with morphine being drip administered to control the aches and pains. That same night, despite being under the influence of pain killers and other drugs, Madeleine found enough strength to call for and converse with her brother Guyto and her mother Thérèse again. These moments when she somehow again communicated with her departed loved ones, were so moving and spiritually powerful that they will be imprinted in my mind for ever. Annabelle woke me up around 2.30 am and told me that *"Meme is having difficulty breathing. She is making strange noises."*

We called the nurse into the room. Despite the removal of fluid from within her lungs and throat, Madeleine passed away at 3.20 am.

Annabelle and I held her hands and comforted her. An amazing thing happened at the very moment she died. Her face and countenance changed from a very stressed and painful look, into one of extreme peace and beauty. We knew immediately that she was not suffering anymore and had crossed the divide between earthly presence and into the 'afterlife'. For some reason, Annabelle and I felt relieved that Madeleine had rejoined her departed loved ones and that the five year battle was over. I closed her eyes, kissed her farewell and made sure that she was comfortable for the last time. Through the grief and emotion I whispered to her: *"I will always love you"*. I then called our sons Gerard and Michel to tell them that Madeleine's suffering was over. I also rang the other loved ones to let them know that Madeleine had left us.

Gerard and Michel with their families and Annabelle's boyfriend Miguel came straightaway to the hospital to say goodbye to Madeleine. I was numbed. It was all over. The spark had gone out of my life and my whole world had fallen apart. My caring, beautiful, loving, supportive, dedicated wife, friend and confidante of 34 years had gone. *"Farewell my darling, I will always love you."*

Chapter 8

The Emptiness without Madeleine

"Take me with you. Let us dance with each other again like we did when we first met. I am still the same and I will always love you." Clancy Philippe

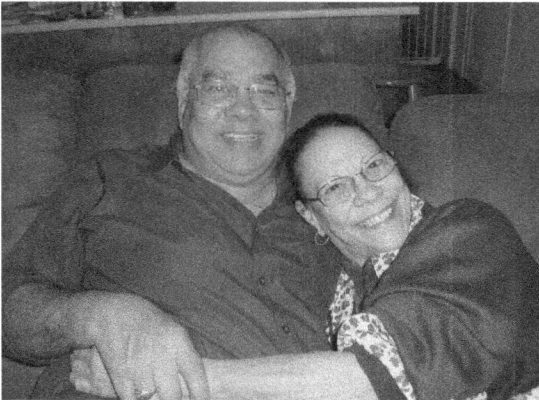

Madeleine and Clancy having cuddles

We stayed at the Cabrini hospital to complete the formalities and left for home, where we all gathered together and offered support and comfort to each other.

I had kissed Madeleine good bye and knew she was now in good hands and re-united with her departed loved ones.

It was strange to be at home and know that Madeleine's smile, laughter and presence would not be there anymore. However, as a family we felt comforted that Madeleine had suffered enough and that she was very much at peace.

As for me, the bottom had fallen out of my world. Life had no more meaning and it was impossible to see how I could face the life ahead of me without her presence at my side. My whole reason for living was gone.

Funeral arrangements had to be made and there were so many other formal and less essential tasks to attend to. My cousin José arranged for me to meet with Father Brian Collins of the Keysborough Resurrection Church to organize the funeral mass. It was my wish that Madeleine would be buried alongside my mother who incidentally shared her name.

The immediate family members were honouring their promise to Madeleine to look after me and along with relatives and friends were there in force, rallying around to make sure I was alright.

I received hundreds of emails from Madeleine's fans worldwide expressing their grief. My mailbox was overflowing. Many would not even accept that Madeleine was not with us anymore.

The messages and phone calls kept pouring in. Visitors came and went. Sympathetic smiles, compassionate hugs and the sharing of stories about Madeleine all found their way into the deep emptiness within my soul. The everyday routine of looking after and caring for Madeleine particularly over the past five years had stopped and absolutely nothing was there to take its place. Through the blur of numbness each and every act of kindness was more appreciated than those who gave them will ever know. I can now thank you from the bottom of my heart for being there for us both.

The contents of these two emails expressed it all:

" I am very sad to hear the news about Madeleine. I did not know her personally but I knew her recipes by heart. I'm a Mauritian who arrived in Sydney two years ago.

With the help of the Website, I learned the traditional recipes of our country. They did bring a lot of joy to me and my husband. Her recipes were to me like an "anti-depression" medicine that helped me get over my home blues in low times.

Thank you to you and Madeleine for that great job. I would like to express my deepest sympathy to you and your family. Bon courage dans ces moments durs de la vie.

Let us think that God needed a little angel by his side to prepare all those lovely dishes and to bring joy up there."

Ian (Dr Ian Haines – Madeleine's long time oncologist and friend) wrote :

"Dear Clancy and family,

I would like you to know how sorry I am about Madeleine's passing. She was a most delightful, positive, determined and courageous lady who coped remarkably well with a terrible illness.

You all did a wonderful job caring for Madeleine and supporting her through this long and difficult time. I know that Madeleine will be very greatly missed by you all. With my very best wishes for your futures – it was a privilege to have known Madeleine and been able to help care for her.

Yours sincerely,

Ian"

Out of the blue, the following poem by an unknown author found its way into my mail box. I adapted it to include a reference to Madeleine's brother Guyto and her Mum Thérèse.

When tomorrow starts without me

And I'm not here to see…
If the sun should rise and find your
Eyes filled with tears for me,
I wish so much you wouldn't cry
The way you did today…
While thinking of the many things
We didn't get to say.
I know how much you love me,
As much as I love you…
And each time you think of me,
I know you'll miss me too.
But when tomorrow starts without me,
Please try to understand…
Jesus, Guyto and Maman came and called my name,
And took my hand.
They said my place was ready
In Heaven far above…
And that I'd have to leave behind
All those I dearly love.
So when tomorrow starts without me,
Don't think we're far apart…
For every time you think of me,
I'm right here in your heart.

~ Adapted from Author Unknown

I woke up each morning and felt the deep void around me. It was hard to explain the loneliness and emptiness that prevailed despite being surrounded by my loved ones and friends. Gerard and the grandsons Brandon and Joshua stayed with me. I looked at them and even though I felt Madeleine's presence through them the devastation and loss was nearly impossible to bear. Living did not make sense anymore. I just did not know how I was going to cope. All I could see was an emptiness ahead.

Chapter 9

Farewell Madeleine and Eulogies

A Eucharistic Celebration thanking God for the life of Madeleine Philippe March 4, 1938 – February 11, 2011

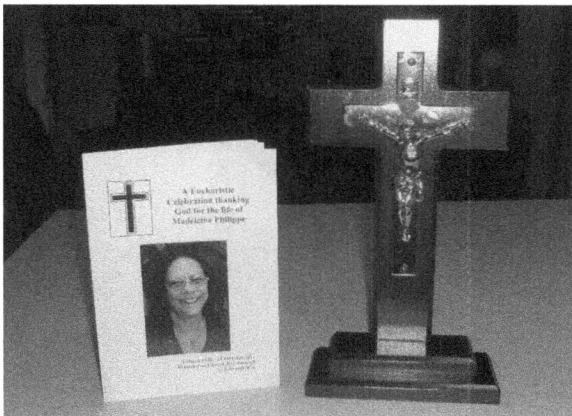

Madeleine's funeral was held at the Resurrection Church in Keysborough, Melbourne on February 17, 2011. It was a farewell to remember, well organised by the Church, the children and grandchildren, in accordance with my wishes. We also displayed a banner celebrating Madeleine's web site *'Recipes from Mauritius'*.

The church was overflowing with relatives, friends, work colleagues and fans of Madeleine. Many had to stand outside the church as all seats and standing room within the church were taken. Some fans travelled interstate to attend the funeral. Father Brian Collins was outstanding in the conduct of the last farewell to Madeleine.

ENTRANCE - Verdi-Slaves Chorus (Nabucco) music, one of Madeleine's favourite choruses by Verdi.
Brandon, Joshua, Jaiden & Nicholas (grandchildren) accompanied Madeleine into the church.

MEMORABILIA - Molly, Joshua, Brandon & Jaiden brought forward memorabilia to remind us of Madeleine and her favourite activities. The memorabilia included a framed photo of Madeleine, a wooden spoon that symbolised Madeleine's culinary passion and the use of same to bring the kids into line, a small bottle of Johnnie Walker (she enjoyed her evening scotch whisky) and a copy of an unfinished crossword magazine.

OPENING PRAYER by Father Brian Collins

LITURGY OF THE WORD, FIRST READING, READING FROM THE BOOK OF WISDOM, RESPONSORIAL PSALM AND GOSPEL read by Diane, Lindy, Reine, Wallis, and Josian.

EULOGIES by Danielle Paruit (Goddaughter), Annabelle deBaize (Granddaughter) on behalf of the grandchildren, Jennifer deBaize (on behalf of Clancy Philippe) and Patrick Morel (on behalf of the Mauritian Community in Melbourne).

HOMILY by Father Brian Collins. This was beautifully presented and deeply touched everybody present.

SONG 'I will always love you' by Whitney Houston. That was my special message to Madeleine.

PRAYERS OF THE FAITHFUL by Jim, Valery, Jean-Pierre & Patrice.

OFFERTORY PROCESSION by Miguel & Doreen.

COMMUNION HYMN Song 'Power of Love'. A message from Madeleine to me. A choice from Heaven.

REFLECTION Song Ave Maria. A traditional Catholic Prayer asking for the intercession of the Virgin Mary. Much loved by Madeleine.

FINAL COMMENDATION AND FAREWELL by Father Brian Collins.

FINAL EXIT Pierre, Jean, Jacques, Josian accompanied Madeleine out of the church.

FINAL HYMN 'Friends for Life' by Brightman & Carreras. A moving message by Madeleine.

We also expressed our thanks to everybody who attended the funeral:

'Madeleine's family would like to sincerely thank you for your kind thoughts, prayers and presence here today. In particular, we wish to thank members of the family and friends who assisted Madeleine & Clancy throughout these difficult times.

Dr Ian Haines and the medical staff at Cabrini Hospital took great care of Madeleine. The City of Greater Dandenong has been very supportive of both Madeleine & Clancy, without whose help Clancy could have never been able to care for Madeleine.'

EULOGIES:

Danielle Paruit:
God daughter and niece of Madeleine.

It has been said that there are two things in life that you can't avoid -Taxes and Death. No matter how creative your accountant, there is no escape from consumption tax.

As for Death, it is the Law of Nature. It is the stage of completion in the Circle of Life, which has its beginning at Birth.

That being said: 'losing someone you love and care for is never easy... no matter how inevitable.' I have known Maddy all of my life – she was my aunt and my godmother, she was my friend.

I was a fortunate child, the first niece in the family, so for a few years monopolised the attention and affection of my father's brothers and sisters. From the very beginning, my relationship with Maddy was one of innate understanding and acceptance of each other's character, full of joy, laughter and respect - that never changed, never vacillated for 52 years.

One of the many characteristics that I most admired about Maddy was her absolute forthrightness and raw honesty. You were never left wondering how she felt or what she was thinking. Although I know that some people may have preferred a more mollycoddled or sanitised approach. This was very much a part of her DNA, no doubt inherited from my grandmother, which I feel that I have also inherited in part… gratefully.

I am sad that Maddy with the toughest of armour had to battle cancer for so many years, only to eventually succumb and surrender.

I am sad that we will no longer share the cackling laughter and unique moments of two people who understand each other, without having to say much.

I am sad that there will no longer be the clinking of the scotch glasses for the ritual of having our trademark photos taken as we have done numerous times over the years.

But I am comforted in my belief that Life here on Earth is merely a stopover. Maddy has transitioned to the next stage of her journey, to join her sister - Miche and brother - Guyto who have had a head start.

I am certain that Maddy's light will shine as brightly at her next destination, as it has here. I'll miss her on a physical level, but I know that she will always be present and never too far away."

Brandon:
Grandson.

"Meme (Madeleine) you have loved us all your life and you have cared for us during the good and the worst you will always be in my heart and you will never be forgotten and everyone loves you lots."

Joshua:
Grandson.

"Every time we see you, it makes our day. But, we couldn't bear to see you suffering in so much pain. It hurt. You are in a better place now where nothing can hurt you anymore. We love you always."

Molly:
Granddaughter.

"From the first day I met Meme, I could see that she was the most amazing woman on the planet. There are so many good memories that I have and are very sacred.

The thing I will never forget is that you didn't get to eat my lasagne as she had to go to hospital. Meme, you will be in my heart forever and always. Rest in Peace. I love you."

Jaiden:
Grandson.

"We cherished and love you. You left us for a better place. We will greatly miss you Meme. Rest in peace Meme. You will always be in my heart."

Annabelle deBaize:
Eldest Granddaughter of Madeleine.

"On behalf of the older grandchildren (Annabelle, Jennifer and Nicholas) I would like to say:

Our Meme was a large influence in our lives. Growing up, we always had strict guidelines that she was certain would turn us into the best people we could be.

We had a certain way to dress, eat at the dinner table, speak and present ourselves when out in public. Meme was a classy woman with excellent manners, dinner etiquette and a fabulous fashion sense just to top off her character. With her gorgeous almost black hair and signature red lipstick and nail polish, you just couldn't miss her coming. Each of us was taught everything she knows. And, if we didn't listen, well, let's just leave it as the wooden spoon was never a friend of ours.

Meme always had faith in God and that faith made her always see the best in people. She would help anybody that needed her help and not hesitate. Her generosity and kindness was passed through to many people, worldwide. She taught us that when you help somebody to never ask for anything in return and do it because you want to do it, not because of what you can get out of it.

Her personality is definitely something we can safely say we all picked up. She was always the first one to tell us exactly how she feels and what she liked or didn't like. I remember one time when I once sat at the dinner table, the tablecloth completely covered my legs. I had them up on the chair crossed and to this day I still have no idea how she knew they were like that. But since that day, I definitely knew better than to do that around her.

She was full of love, energy and no matter what, she was always there for her family. She was always proud of us and pushing us to become something great when we grew up. She always encouraged our education and told us that there wasn't anything we couldn't do. Her family always came first.

She was always cooking for us, always cleaning up after our mess even though she wanted to kill us, always being kind and gentle when she needed to be there for us and definitely not scared to teach us a lesson knowing we would be better people for it. She was always proud of everything we accomplished and she was never shy to show it.

She was the heart of our family. She is our hero. We are so thankful for everything she did for us. She is somebody we all want to become. With her in our life and in our hearts, we can achieve anything we set our minds to. She is the wind beneath our wings.

Our Meme has been there from the moment each of us was born, to this day and she will forever be with us. We love you Meme, we will miss you and wait for the day we can all be reunited as the great family you built."

Clancy Philippe:
Husband of Madeleine - read by Jennifer deBaize.

"I first laid eyes on you some 37 years ago and was captured by your smile and magnetic personality. That was love at first sight. Three years later, we were married and that was the beginning of the best 34 years of my life. The two of us became one. You always knew how I felt and I always knew how you felt. You spent the rest of your life totally dedicated to me and the family. In return, I made sure that no harm ever came to you.

Five years ago, you were struck with breast cancer. We rallied together we fought hard. You won that first battle and we went on a world tour, during which time you blossomed and were radiant in happiness. These seven weeks were the best time we had together, visiting relatives, friends and places that you told me you had never been to.

Fate struck again and you were diagnosed with ovarian cancer. Again we rallied and fought hard. We won, only to be struck again with secondary breast cancer, followed by secondary ovarian cancer. That was our last battle together. We fought hard and tough. But your body was tired and gave up the fight. Your mind and spirit still urged you to keep fighting, but you had no fight left in you.

You had suffered enough already. I was helpless and could do nothing to help you. It hurt so bad when you said to me in hospital: "Help me !" and I could do nothing. But you fought on and lost the battle on the morning of February 11th. I have not only lost my darling wife, but also my lifelong best friend.

Half of me is going away, but half of you is staying in me. The happy memories live on and I am the luckiest man alive as you gave me the best 34 years of my life. Thank you for looking after me so well. I was never wanting for anything.

Farewell my Louloune and I know that from Paradise, you will still be looking after me and your loved ones. Farewell and take care until we meet again. Most importantly, I will always love you.

I wish to thank the family and friends who cared for Madeleine during these difficult times. I wish to thank Dr Ian Haines and the Cabrini nursing staff who took such great care of Madeleine.

Also, a big thank you to the City of Greater Dandenong for their understanding, assistance and help. They supported me in giving the best care possible to Madeleine.

Thank you all for being present today."

Patrick Morel:
On behalf of the Mauritian Community in Melbourne.

"My dear friends, it is very comforting to see how the community has assembled here today to celebrate the life of Maddy as tributes from here and many countries keep flowing in.

The Press at home was very prompt in offering their respects to a special Lady. In spite of all the sadness that we feel, the family in particular, let's remind ourselves that this is no final curtain.

It is a celebration of the life of a much loved member of the community who was so dynamic and contributed so much to the wellbeing of the Mauritian Diaspora. Not only in Australia, Melbourne in particular but in many more countries through the link of the dedicated website maintained by Clancy and accessed by all Mauritians worldwide 24 hours a day permanently.

Accessed also by non-Mauritians who have been introduced to our delicacies by the recipes written or verified and endorsed by Maddy, always respecting the original concepts.

Maddy displayed an incredible resilience in the face of adversity and put on the bravest face whilst enjoying life and the company of her legions of friends in the community. My niece shared a table in the company of Boum and Maddy at a year-end party, and when I gave her the sad news, she did not think it possible. My niece did not know the circumstances and thought that Maddy was the life of the party.

After visiting Melbourne in the seventies and being captivated, the family settled here in the early 80s. Soon the website was created to highlight the marvels that delight our taste buds. And the world started visiting, tasting and sharing.

Daily visits have grown from an early 1500 daily to 4500 on average now. Yesterday, 6363 clicked on the site. On the record too, these visitors came from 45 countries and more. That's an example of the friends attracted to the delights that Maddy and Clancy disseminated for our taste buds.

Her activities, although dominated by Mauritian cuisine, included writing about Mauritian cuisine in such high profile publications as the Lonely Planet Travel Guide, taking part in club activities and creating cancer awareness among friends and relatives via the *'Madeleine Philippe Cancer Foundation (Aus) Inc'*.

Wherever she went, she would always be discussing cooking techniques with other people during her travels, adding more credits to her experience.

Hobbies were essentially looking after Mr. Boum and the family, children, grand children, daughters in law and unending groups of friends.

The website received many rewards and recognitions. Nowadays it stands proudly as a world leader in its field and an essential connection for the Mauritian Diaspora worldwide. Maddy's name is a reference in itself.

Clancy will push forward her dream of publishing a book on genuine Mauritian Multicultural Cuisine in a class of its own. Her recipes will be forever present in people's homes through the magic of the book and the internet.

Her recipes and many more that have not been published yet will be forthcoming.

Clancy has made this a priority.

Five years ago unfortunately, illness raised its ugly head, Maddy fought with determination and courage. Maddy is leaving as a testament to others the Foundation bearing her name. It will keep going, fully dedicated to helping, comforting others.

Whilst offering our condolences to Clancy and the family, it must be noted that at this moment, Maddy is busy at work. All around her, including the big bosses, up there in Heaven, have big smiles lighting up their faces.

The great news is that the impossible is possible.

Up there in Heaven, THE MENU IS CHANGING – FOR THE BETTER - BON APPÉTIT"

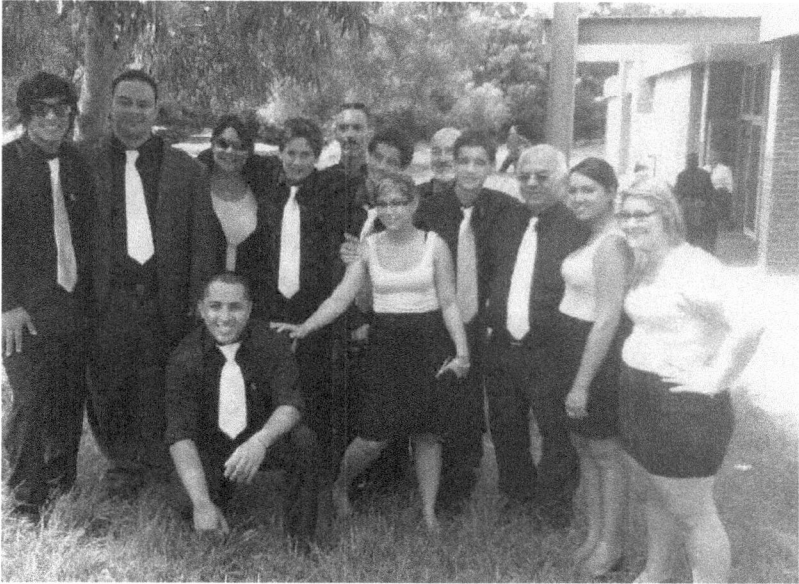

The loved ones after the Farewell to Madeleine
dressed in pink and black for breast cancer

Marcel Lindsay Noë: *A very good friend of the family who sent this from Mauritius.*

"Like the flame on her stove, she silently and gradually faded away after having shared her dreams with loved ones and friends whether near or in faraway places, linked together by the worldwide web woven by the love of her life, her companion on earth, her devoted husband Clancy.

After an epic battle against the illness that blunted her spirited enjoyment of life for so long, she bowed out when God's hands touched her and signalled to her that she will suffer no more and that she will now rejoice in eternal peace in God's Kingdom.

She is not present on this earth anymore but her spirit lives on and will always be present in our kitchens when we will call upon her culinary expertise, that she so passionately shared with all her friends and lovers of Mauritian cuisine worldwide.

She has now rejoined her sister Miche with whom she shared the same 'joie de vivre', the same resonant laughter. I am sure that from the heavenly clouds among the angels, they will be watching us and smiling at our culinary stumbles when we somehow miss Madeleine's special touch in the preparation of those favourite dishes that she could so expertly put together with her eyes closed.

Farewell Maddy. You will be in our hearts forever…and without doubt very much alive in our taste buds. Je t'embrasse, fort. Très fort."

Lindsay (Marcel Lindsay Noë)

Irlande Alfred: *Poem from good friend of Madeleine and Clancy.*

Let Us Celebrate Madeleine

My friends,
Let us not mourn Madeleine
Let us celebrate her life so well lived!

Let us celebrate the happiness and love that
Madeleine shared with us all,

Let us celebrate her 'joie de vivre'.
Let us celebrate her passion for Mauritian Cuisine,

Let us be inspired by her example,
Always in the forefront
To welcome, to love.

Let the recipes from Madeleine
And the happy memories of the time spent together
Comfort us.

Irlande

Mary Dallas:
Email from one of Clancy's colleague at the City of Greater Dandenong.

"Hi my friend

I feel privileged to have attended your lady's farewell which highlighted her great attributes and the unique bond you shared!

As I have previously said to you, consider yourself blessed to have found your soul mate and to have spent so many wonderful years together!

It was a lovely service with very special effects – music and photos – which only you with Madeleine's inspiration could have put together! Another success story by Clancy and Madeleine!

There is no doubt that your lady's memory will live on as she has touched so many hearts and influenced so many lives!

Take care and come back to us when ready!

Warmest thoughts

Mary Dallas"

Doreen M:

Madeleine's ex-daughter in law.

"I am sure Maddy was there in spirit and will be eternally thankful to have had such a husband like you as you loved her unconditionally and would do anything possible for her.

Her send off was beautifully done and as you stated the funeral mass was so meaningful that it really opened my eyes about the whole dying thing. Hence me accepting Maddy no longer being with us but it certainly doesn't mean that I won't miss her.

She has been a mother to me in the 22 years that I have known her and I will eternally be thankful for all the good things she has taught me.

You will always be in my heart Maddy and I know that you will be there to guide me as always so it's not Goodbye it's See u Soon.

All my love until we meet again.

Doreen"

Media:

The newspapers in Mauritius and the Australian Mauritian-Community radios broadcasted the sad news of Madeleine's passing. The 'Le Mauricien' newspaper in Mauritius published the following:

Farewell to Madeleine Philippe, the Queen of Mauritian Cuisine.

"Madeleine Philippe, the smiling lady with the thousand recipes, that delighted lovers of Mauritian Cuisine worldwide, lost her fight with breast and ovarian cancers on February 11, 2011. After a five year long and courageous battle against this dreadful disease, Madeleine Philippe, née Paruit, passed away at 3.23 am (Australian Eastern Time) on Friday morning, in Melbourne where she lived. Her funeral will be held on Thursday February 17, at the Resurrection Church on Corrigan Road in Keysborough at 10.00 am. Her web site http://ile-maurice.tripod.com is the world renowned internet reference on Mauritian Cuisine that receives in excess of 4500 visits daily.

Madeleine Philippe has on many occasions been interviewed on her love for cooking by numerous newspapers and magazines, including Le Mauricien and Week-End/Scope.

Mauritian by birth, she was born in Quatre Bornes and was the librarian of the Carnegie Library in Curepipe for many years.

At the tender age of fifteen, she was initiated into the secrets of Mauritian cuisine. She used her imaginative culinary mind to put together special creations for the enjoyment of family and friends.

She had a flying start with the help of her mother Thérèse (née Latapie), her elder brothers and Masterchef Philippe Auleebux, a close and esteemed friend of the family. Inventive in her approach, Madeleine Philippe would surprise her guests with her special touch that transformed simple dishes into culinary masterpieces. Her passion knew no limits.... She went as far as visiting the kitchen of the famous Rio Restaurant in Curepipe, with Philippe Auleebux, to learn the secrets of Chinese cuisine from the very best.

In the 1980's she migrated to Australia, the lucky country. With her husband and the family, she settled in the State of Victoria and later into the most beautiful city in the world, Melbourne. The internet provided a wonderful opportunity to promote the secrets of Mauritian cuisine. With her husband Clancy in 1994, Madeleine Philippe established the first websites on the internet promoting Mauritius and its cuisine.

The *'Mauritius Australia Connection'* website incorporating the *'Recipes from Australia'* web site now receives in excess of 4500 visits daily from the Mauritian community in Australia and worldwide. Madeleine and Clancy Philippe also laid the foundation for the Madeleine Philippe Cancer Foundation (Aus) Inc to promote the early detection of breast and ovarian cancers."

Chapter 10

Let me tell you about Madeleine

"Let me tell you about Madeleine."

The shock is easing off but the pain is still there with the highs and lows. I alternate between acceptance and downright grief asking myself: *"Why her and why me?"* One minute I am all cheery and the next minute, tears are streaming uncontrollably when I flashback to the happy times we had together. In church last Sunday, tears were streaming down my cheeks at the thought of her not being around anymore.

Grief drives you to feel like you are lifeless with no incentive to do or start doing anything. However, when I think of Madeleine, she would not want me to let go and be miserable. So I recompose myself and get going again. She was not one to let go and I remember the good times we had together and her support for all things that I wanted to achieve.

We had more than a great marriage. Some people called it a 'Love story'. Many referred to us as the perfect couple. The two individuals merged into one entity.

She knew me perfectly and I knew her perfectly. We daily exchanged our thoughts on things that took place during the day. No important decision was ever made without an exchange of opinion on our personal views. After 34 years of marriage, we were still in love like 17 years old teenagers. She loved me unconditionally and I loved her unconditionally. We were best friends and thrived on one another's company; we kept in touch with each other at all times. I remember when on one of the rare occasions that she travelled overseas without me, the phone bill was greater than a return air fare to where she was. That did not matter as we had to know what each other was doing at all times.

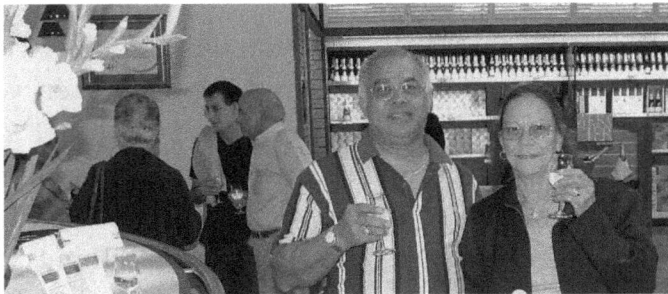

Madeleine and Clancy in Epernay, France

One incident stands out in my mind about Madeleine and how much she valued the importance of life-work balance, even before those words became the subject of constant debate.

One Friday afternoon in Mauritius, we returned from work and I opened the car boot to carry some fifty work files into the house. I had some catch up work to do. Madeleine looked at me and she said: *"If you take this into the house and spend the weekend working, I am going away for the weekend."* No need to tell you that the work files found their way back into the car boot faster than I took them out. That was Madeleine at her best, protecting the welfare of her loved ones. I will miss her caring. For her, the family was at the very top of her priorities.

When anyone asks me about Madeleine, I always tell them that she was one of a kind and the perfect partner. Her mission in life was to make sure that I was never wanting for anything and that the family was OK. In return, I made sure that she was not wanting for anything and that no harm came to her. On top of it all, she was classy without being obnoxious. A kind of subtle classiness that made sure that good manners, good dress sense, respect for others and considerate behaviour prevailed. She was forthright in her views and left you in no doubt as to what her thoughts were.

Every morning, I would leave home for work and kiss her good bye. She would make sure that I was dressed properly and would remind me to be careful on the road both to and from work.

Every evening, she would welcome me with a welcome kiss and tell me about her day. One of her most important tasks was to feed me well and make sure that I had the best meals that could ever be cooked.

When I asked her last Christmas and for her birthday *"What would you like?"* she responded by saying *"I have everything and there is really nothing that I particularly want."* I gave her the same answer on similar occasions. We generally agreed to something that would be of common interest or something that that one of us would really want to have. That's how we bought an iPad in December last and that was her last present to me. Of course, we both prayed for her health to come back.

Losing Madeleine was what I feared most in life, but I didn't see it coming despite her long term battle with breast, ovarian, secondary breast cancer and metastatic ovarian cancer. She would win one battle after another and despite her worsening condition during her last two months, I was used to her battling her way through. It hurt real badly when she was in hospital with only days to live.

She said to me: *"Please help me"* and there was nothing I could do. So far, I had been able to fix things for her every time, all the time. Cancer had me beaten this time.

We all know something about grief and loss. When someone is diagnosed with cancer, we go through a grieving process: the death of our former selves, followed by finding our new normal. That's what Madeleine and I did, although this time I'm grieving her death and the end of my life with her, and finding my new normal without her. Grieving the loss of Madeleine has been the hardest thing I've ever done. Every now and then, I cry uncontrollably and beg God to help me through this pain. Missing Madeleine and not being able to do anything about it, except linger in this achingly slow passage of time is agonizing. With the support of the loved ones, I realize that while it doesn't seem like it, I am beginning to slowly move forward. I am moving through some of this pain and grief. Half of me has gone with her but half of her has stayed with me.

I take comfort that Madeleine was respected and loved by all. Messages of condolence poured from all over the world and the church overflowed with loved ones, family, friends and work colleagues during her funeral service. *"Caring, sincere and loving"* were some of the words I heard over and over to describe her; she did things because they were the right things to do, and so many people told me how much they loved her. She was a person who put God, loved ones, family, friends and doing the right thing above all else.

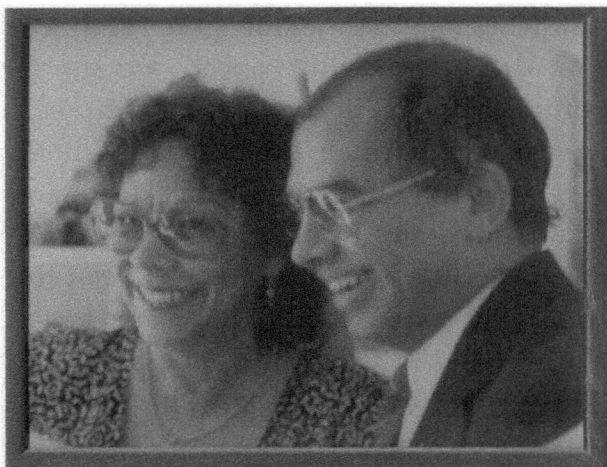

"Madeleine (or Louloune as I called her), I will always love you, need you, want you, miss you and marvel at you. I know you are with God. Please call and let me know you got there alright."

Chapter 11

Looking for a Reason to Live

"There's a love that only you can give, a smile that only your lips can show, a twinkle that can only be seen in your eyes and my life that only you can complete." Anon

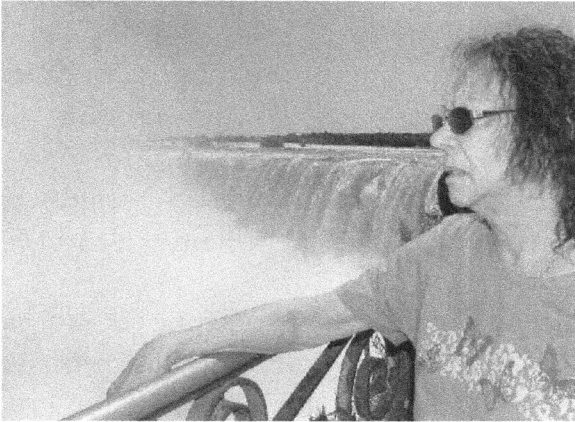

Madeleine at Niagara Falls

Not that my attitude to life was flawed. I considered myself to be reasonably well balanced before Madeleine's departure. Madeleine's loss made many of life's little problems and issues unimportant in the overall scheme of things.

One outcome of all this very painful and sad experience is that *"I am not scared of death anymore"* and if I was told tomorrow that I had some incurable disease and only had months to live, I would be comfortable with that. There is someone waiting for me on the other side of the divide.

The support from people that I never had any contact with before was phenomenal. It was truly amazing to find that there was so much love for Madeleine and how much she had contributed to people's happiness in many ways.

I was touched by the outpouring of grief from friends and strangers alike and I will always treasure the words contained in the many messages sent in the months after her death. The sentiments expressed became my lifeline and gave me great strength to pull myself together.

I received this email from someone I had never met before. It expressed beautifully how much Madeleine has stayed in me, will never go and is destined to last forever.

"Dear Clancy,

Your story brought tears to my eyes, and tears are still streaming from my eyes as I write this message to you. First off, I would like to express my deepest, heartfelt sympathy to you and your family for the passing of Madeleine.

However, I do not feel that you have lost her at all. She's very much around you because the two of you are Soul Mates - thus, you are inseparable throughout eternity.

I'm not sure what I can really say to ease your pain (even a little); but from what I understand about Soul Mates is that only a very small percentage of people ever get to meet and/or marry their Soul Mate. You and Madeleine beat the odds by not only meeting and marrying each other, but also sharing many blissful years together. Please understand that this is a divine gift and blessing from God.

The two of you shared a very rare love - unconditional love. Somehow, God felt that the two of you were deserving of this wonderful gift and blessing. So please try to see it for what it is. So many people go through life not finding their own souls, let alone their Soul Mate. They live their lives on auto pilot and with blinkers on.

I believe that Madeleine is very much with you and watching over you right now. Your souls are still entwined and always will be.

My hope is that you will share your beautiful love story with the world, because if there's one thing we all need to learn is 'unconditional love' and service to one another. Please tell the world what a real relationship and marriage is all about so humanity can raise its consciousness.

And don't worry about getting writer's block - Madeleine will help you with this. I think it will not only help to keep her beautiful memory alive, but it will further remind you that, although her physical body is no longer with us, her soul is very much alive.

I am looking forward to purchasing a copy of this book should you ever decide to write it. I also look forward to someday meeting and marrying my own Soul Mate. May God bless you and your family - and may God bless Madeleine.

Sincerely,
Elizabeth Ducasse"

Another email from a school friend with whom I have kept in touch and he knew Madeleine quite well. He had also lost his wife to cancer only the year before.

"Dear Boum,

It is with a heavy heart that I received the sad news. Please accept my sincere condolences to you and your close ones. The road ahead may be rough, but you can rest assured that my thoughts will be with you, if only to lighten your steps in some little way.

Maddy has been cheery and strong and she will surely wish that you be so.

I am now in Hong Kong, on my way alone to Mauritius before going back to China. Thierry, Denys and I are just back from China, where I took them to visit the family place and meet some relatives, which is a duty I felt necessary to be fulfilled. I trust they had a memorable time during this short first stay.

Brothers in laughter, we are now brothers in sorrow. When shared, the former is multiplied and the latter gets lighter. May our friendship stand the test of time and support you at this time of bereavement. My ears and my door are always open to you.
Hugs, Chin."

The following email is from someone who had known Madeleine through meeting her at community functions.

"Dear Clancy,

This is sad news – I am very sorry to hear this.

Madeleine has been an inspiration to us all. The times I have met her, she beamed with a radiance that is so unique. She clearly has given this world a lot and she is a lady that can provide us with inspiration and hope.

Her efforts in the Mauritian community have been excellent and such that many can learn from.

On behalf of myself and the team at Air Mauritius please know that our thoughts are with you and your family. If we can help in any way, please do not hesitate to let me know.

Please keep in touch.
Steven P."

This next email came from Father Pierre Piat.

"Dear Clancy,

I am thinking of you following the passing of Madeleine. Her departure must leave a great void in your life. I can assure you of my love and brotherly prayers during this very difficult time.

She was very gifted and the happy memories of her will lead to our 'Thanksgiving' for the way she contributed to our happiness.

Yours affectionately,
Father Pierre Piat"

Another email came from one of her fans.

"Madeleine was an extraordinary woman who has done so much for Mauritian cuisine, thanks to her and the Philippe's website those recipes are now known worldwide, she should be an inspiration to others. May she rest in peace. God bless"

Marianne M."

There were days when not even the sentiments in the messages could lift me in the darkest and lowest point in my life. Alone with just my thoughts, I felt the utter despair and began to understand why sometimes people consider ending their lives as a serious option. I felt that way many times as my life was empty without her. Somehow, that would have been one way for me to be with her again. Common sense prevailed and watching how much I was loved by my loved ones, caring friends and Madeleine's fans worldwide, I realized that I was very lucky to have so much support and affection. Many people in the same situation have nothing.

I was somehow logical in my thinking. I analysed the situation like all engineers do and concluded that I was heading for the precipice of depression or something similar. I could not see the light at the end of the tunnel. I had been dealt a fatal blow with no apparent hope of recovery. The slightest thought of Madeleine made me cry.

My eyes were almost permanently clouded with tears and I constantly had to rush to the box of tissues. My outside displayed strength and resilience. Inside I was crumbling like a building that was on the verge of collapse. The only thought that kept me going was that Madeleine would never accept that I was giving up.

The uncanny thought conversation that I started to have with Madeleine urged me to collect myself and move forward. The sight of her smile brought me back to my senses and urged me not to quit. If ever, I were to recover, it would be for Madeleine as she gave me the strength to keep going.

By then, I started releasing my feelings and despair into writing this book. This decision had been taken whilst Madeleine was still alive and she knew that I was going to write about our encounter with cancer and how this dreadful disease takes over your life. Our aim was to offer support to people who suffer from cancer, assist loved ones battling cancer or are recovering from the trauma of losing loved ones to cancer. We always discussed our projects and she was totally supportive of this one. *'The worst part of holding the memories is not the pain. It's the loneliness of it. Memories need to be shared.'* — *Lois Lowry in The Giver.* That was another reason why I started writing to share the memories of it all with others.

Meanwhile, some strange events started happening. One night, some two weeks after Madeleine's funeral, I was awakened and felt like I was looking down at the bed in which I was sleeping.

I could see myself in bed and beside me was a body shape of the same size as Madeleine's. Initially, I thought it was my grandson Brandon who was in the guest bedroom. I asked twice: *"Is that you Brandon?"* It was 2.13 am and that body shape stayed beside me for what appeared to be 30 seconds or so. I did not say anything to anyone and put it down to some sort of a dream.

Since Madeleine's passing, I have been very meticulous in making up the bed every morning, taking great care to fold the bed sheet, organize the pillows and place the doona cover on top very carefully, so as not to make it apparent that half the bed was empty. One morning, I woke up to find the bedcover corner on Madeleine's side flipped over as if someone was getting into bed. The bed cover was fairly heavy and there was no way in my sleep that I could have folded it over the way it was. Again, I paid little attention to this and only briefly mentioned it to other people.

Late one Saturday morning. I went into the bedroom to get something. When I walked in, there was a very strong smell of Madeleine's favourite perfume.

It was as if Madeleine had just entered the bedroom, except that the smell was stronger.

I checked to see if I had spilt some of Madeleine's perfume, but all her perfume bottles were in their right places in her perfume basket. Nothing spilt. The perfume smell lasted for a few minutes, and then it was gone.

I started asking myself questions. *'Am I hallucinating'* or *'Have I lost my marbles'*. It was more than that and my cousin Jose reminded me how at Madeleine's funeral in the Church of Resurrection in Keysborough, there was a problem with the incense burner. The incense burner was left unlit in the church mass preparation room. During the funeral service, when it was time to light up the charcoal in the burner it would not light up. Multiple unsuccessful attempts were tried by several people to get the charcoal to burn. As soon as Madeleine's coffin was taken from the church into the hearse, the incense charcoal started to burn so brightly that it had to be extinguished for fear of burning everything around it. We all remembered that Madeleine could not stand the smell of incense.

During the night of April 2, 2011, I dreamt of Madeleine. She was dressed in one of her 'kaftan' style dresses and looked fresh and much younger. The environment was an extremely green, beautiful and bright natural landscape.

I was following her and she had an unlit cigarette in one hand and was carrying a brown bag in the other. I remember clearly saying to her: *"You have not started smoking again!"* She did not answer me, but kept on walking. We arrived at the foreshore of a wide river with very clear flowing water and a group of young looking 'old people' on the rocky banks of the river. Among them, I recognized one of our old friends who died some 15 years ago. It was Philippe Auleebux, the same guy with whom Madeleine shared a passion for Mauritian cuisine. I told Annabelle about this dream and she asked: *"Meme (Madeleine) was carrying a brown bag!"* I answered yes. She went into her room and came back saying: *"Meme gave me this bag a long time ago."* It was exactly the same brown bag. How do you explain this incredible coincidence?

At the funeral, we played the songs *"I Will Always Love You"* and *"The Power of Love"*. These were like my last messages to Madeleine. On April 3, 2011, on my way to visit Madeleine at the Botanical Gardens Cemetery in Springvale, I was very down and begged Madeleine to be in touch with me again after the dream I had had the night before. On my way up a new overpass to the EastLink Freeway, I suddenly thought of John Denver. He had never known true love, whereas my true love was gone. I switched on the car radio and could not believe my ears.

The song "For You" by John Denver was being played and despite being a John Denver fan, I had never heard this song before. Even stranger was the fact that the channel broadcasting the song was one I rarely listened to and yet for some reason I had selected this particular station as I was driving along.

The tears flowed as I listened to the words, but was left in no doubt that this was all Madeleine's doing and was her way of responding to my cry for help:

"Just to wake up each morning
Just to you by my side
Just to know that you're never really far away
Just a reason for living
Just to say I adore
Just to know that you're in my heart to stay"

Words from *"Just You"* by John Denver.

This incident was a turning point in the downward spiral. From that moment on I had this strong feeling that Madeleine was watching over me and was never far away. She was giving me a reason for living again.

Around the same time, I started downloading and reading eBooks written by others about their loved ones' battles with cancer. Lo and behold, in the second book that I read, someone wrote about her walking into a late friend's home and smelling the lavender perfume that her friend loved to wear.

Same scenario, the smell disappeared after a few minutes. In the book, the writer spoke about this perfume smell making its appearance on more than a few occasions, in very similar circumstances to mine.

Before Madeleine's departure, I had an open mind about these things. And being an engineer by profession, I needed the facts before I could support the belief held by some people, especially of the older generation, that these things happen and result from our departed loved ones communicating with us after death. I researched the subject and was slowly seeing things from a different perspective.

It was not because I was reading about it or people were convincing me that there was life after death. Strange things were happening to me which were as real as anything I had experienced before. They defied logic and normal comprehension and were taking place in my life for the very first time. My engineering expertise and logic were seriously challenged.

Madeleine on the other hand, was indeed giving me a reason to live again.

Chapter 12

Near and After-Death Communications

"On the other side I felt really good and found spiritual tranquility and supreme peacefulness." Guyto Paruit - Madeleine's brother on his 'After-Death Experience'.

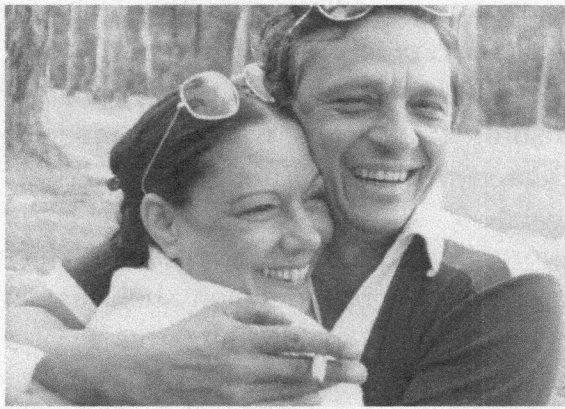

Madeleine and brother Guyto – inseparable siblings

I researched the subject of near and after-death communications and numerous true stories emerged. Olivia Newton-John recalls this ghostly experience just after her mother died.

Sitting alone with the body of her mother, Olivia Newton-John felt 'an incredible presence' in the room. *"It was an energy I'd never felt before,"* the singer said. Recalling a conversation the pair had some time earlier, she asked her mum to send a signal that she was OK wherever she was now. *"Make the candles move, or flicker, or something,"* Olivia urged. Some small candles in the room moved a little, enough to reassure her. But then she was called to the living room where family and friends were gathered. *"You'll never believe what happened,"* they said. A candle in that room had just exploded with a fizzing sound right under the picture of Olivia's mother. The incident is among a collection of stories of the supernatural in a new book *'The Dying Experience and Learning How to Live.'* by Mike Agostini. This story was first made public on Andrew Denton's TV show 'Enough Rope.'

Another story involved Olympic gold medal swimmer Dawn Fraser and happened when she was seriously ill with glandular fever soon after giving birth to her daughter. *"I really felt I was going to die,"* she said. *"Suddenly I saw what looked like my late father's face on my wardrobe. Get out of bed, Dawny,"* he said. 'The next morning I again saw his profile and heard the words, *"Get out of bed, Dawny. So I got up."* If I hadn't seen that profile and heard those words, I would have died.'

In 2003, the head of the United Nations office in Australia, Juan Carlos Brandt, spoke at a memorial service for officers and staff who had been killed by a bomb in Baghdad. Agostini, writer on after-death communication was present and commented on how the wind rose strongly when the names of those who had died were read, Brandt looked at him intensely and said: *"That wasn't the only thing. I could distinctly hear Nadia's voice"* (Nadia was a senior secretary and close friend of Brandt's who was killed by the bomb). *"Even above the wind, I could hear her saying, Piss off, Juan Carlos! We're all right, all of us. You get on with your work and do what you have to do because we're OK."*

In 1994, the surviving former members of The Beatles - Paul McCartney, George Harrison, and Ringo Starr - got together to record 'Free As a Bird', a song written by Lennon before his death. During the recording session, paranormal experiences were reported. *"There were a lot of strange goings-on in the studio - noises that shouldn't have been there and equipment doing all manner of weird things,"* Paul McCartney said. *"There was just an overall feeling that John was around."*

In 2007, Lennon's son, Julian, said he was contacted by the ghost of his late father. At the time, Julian was taking part in a traditional Australian Aboriginal ceremony when a tribal leader handed him a white feather.

Julian found this highly significant since John had told him that if he should ever die to be vigilant for the gift of a white feather. It would mean that he was present and looking out for him.

As the wacky red-headed 'Queen of Comedy', Lucille Ball enjoyed a long career on TV with her shows *I Love Lucy*, *The Lucy-Desi Comedy Hour*, *The Lucy Show* and *Here's Lucy*. Lucy's ghost may still be getting into trouble at her Beverly Hills home on Roxbury Drive. Those who have lived there since her passing have reported loud voices in the attic, furniture being rearranged and even unexplained broken windows. Lucy is also thought to haunt the building that served as DesiLu Studios on the Paramount lot where night watchmen have reported a female ghost on the upper floor who gives off a perfumed scent.

Heath Ledger was one of the most promising actors of his generation, having delivered impressive performances in such films as *Brokeback Mountain* and *The Dark Knight*, in which his portrayal of The Joker drew wide acclaim. He died in January, 2008 of what was ruled an accidental overdose of sleeping pills. Actress Michelle Williams, his ex-fiancé, says she has seen Ledger's spirit on two occasions. The first time, she was awakened at night by eerie noises, then realized her bedroom furniture was being moved around.

She saw a shadowy figure, which she admits scared her 'half to death'. In the second instance, she says the apparition was much more vivid and spoke, telling her he was sorry for not being able to help raise their daughter.

In a previous chapter I wrote about being present when Madeleine sat up on her death bed, and reached out for her dead mother Thérèse, despite being in a coma and unable to move. She also had numerous conversations with her brother Guyto who died in 2007. I also told you about the corner of my bedcover being flipped over, the smell of Madeleine's favourite perfume in the bedroom and the presence of a body shape in bed beside me. These paranormal events led me to open up my mind about events for which I could not find any 'earthly' explanations.

In '*The Australian Weekend Australian Magazine*' on May 21, 2011 Kate Legge wrote about near-death conversations with departed loved ones.

"Not everyone near to death reports seeing or sensing the presence of relatives who have gone before them. "You'd best ask the cleaners what they hear," jokes Deborah O'Connor, 53, a former palliative care nurse in the Newcastle region who has watched "hundreds of people die". She believes patients are more likely to reveal visions to a worker with a broom than a doctor in a white coat.

Her first glimpse into death's secrets occurred in an oncology ward during her early 20s. "There was a young man who had died in the room with his family and I saw an aura coming off him. It was like a mist. I didn't tell anybody for years. I've never seen it again." Researching her Master's thesis on this subject, she spoke to two nurses who were in a room with a patient's husband when they all observed the same 'aura'.

Familiar with the spectrum of possibilities that may distinguish a death, she rattles off things she has encountered. "Most commonly people tell me they have seen dead relatives. Families will come to us and say, 'Joe's saying his mother came to see him, but his mother died 20 years ago.'

I have seen, and nurses have reported to me, patients doing things they haven't been able to do for weeks, like sitting bolt upright in bed with a sudden super-consciousness. Sometimes they might say things like, 'I'm coming.' Patients may wait until a loved one gets there before dying and sometimes they choose to die only after somebody special to them has left the room," she says.

Now health promotion officer with La Trobe University's palliative care unit, O'Connor urges nurses to accept these events as a normal occurrence. "Families often find it distressing. They think the patient is out of control, hallucinating.

If they understand these things are quite common it settles everyone down," she says. "The point I make is that if a dying person says it's happened, then it's real for them. I don't think people go around making these things up. They're dying. They've got nothing to lose."

I came across the book 'Reflections of a Setting Sun' by Dr Michael Barbaro (a medical practitioner who now specializes in after-death experiences and has undertaken considerable research in the subject).

When Dr Barbato first began writing about these phenomena in the late '90s he was regarded as 'very fringe'. Now he tours the country addressing conferences of doctors, nurses and palliative care staff. He said *"People who once thought I'd lost my marbles are now prepared to listen."*

After-death Communication (Extract from 'Reflections of a Setting Sun' by Dr Michael Barbato):

"Following the death of a loved one, it is not uncommon for a bereaved relative, usually the spouse or partner, to sense the presence of the deceased person. This sensation may be so indistinct the bereaved person dismisses it or suspects their mind is playing tricks. More often than not, however, the experience is so strong the person rarely doubts its validity – it feels too real not to be true.

The experience may be one off or many and varied. They tend to occur in the first weeks - months following the death and often during periods of solitude and stillness. For this reason they are more common when the person is alone, last thing at night, first thing in the morning or while resting. They can, however, happen at the most unlikely times e.g. while showering or while driving the car. The nature of the experience varies, but most commonly involves one or more of the following:

- *a sense of the deceased person being close by*

- *a feeling of being touched, stroked or held*

- *hearing their voice*

- *smelling their perfume or aftershave*

- *seeing the deceased person*

- *a profound dream featuring the deceased*

- *a synchronistic event such as hearing the deceased person's favourite song/piece of music played on the radio on their birthday, anniversary, etc.*

When I first started work as a palliative care doctor, I was surprised when the occasional grieving relative told me about their experiences.

I then started to ask around and was not only surprised by the number who had an after-death experience but also by the relief they felt in talking about it and having the experience validated.

The experience, as bizarre as it may seem, is almost always comforting, even though the person is frequently overcome by emotion. Most treasure the experience, yet they are often reluctant to talk about it for fear it will be dismissed or that they will be misjudged. On this point it should be noted that those who have such an experience are NOT insane or imagining things. What they experience is undeniably real to them and, as incomprehensible as it may seem to others, their account of events should not be doubted, downplayed or disrespected.

After-death experiences were once considered 'abnormal', but are now believed to be a normal and healthy part of the grieving process occurring in up to 50% of surviving spouses/partners. There are numerous theories concerning their origin ranging from the psychological to the transcendental with the weight of evidence favouring a rational explanation rather than a metaphysical cause.

Despite this, many, if not most who have an after-death experience are convinced their deceased relative is trying to communicate an important message. This message is rarely expressed in words but is understood at an intuitive level.

It may be a message of love or a final good-bye, but always there is a reassuring undertone to indicate they (the deceased) are okay. Once the message is realised it is not uncommon for the communication to cease.

On rare occasions the communication has a utilitarian dimension and in these cases the message, while still implicit, has a little more detail. For example, one person described how her recently deceased husband 'told' her where to locate an item that she, and the rest of the family, had searched for in vain. Another said her deceased husband had appeared to their son-in-law, asking him to take care of the family. These matter-of-fact messages are (not surprisingly) more often communicated by men.

Accounts of after-death experiences are compelling, and the air of mystery that surrounds them continues to fuel the ongoing debate as to whether there is life after death. Science suggests after-death communication does not arise from disembodied beings but from the psyche of the bereaved. However, many of the bereaved that I have spoken to say, that as a result of their experience, they now believe in eternal life. Some were previously non-believers, but the convincing nature of the experience or the significant message contained therein has forever changed their opinion. In time we shall all experience death; only then will the truth be revealed."

Chapter 13

More Visits by Madeleine

"The beginning of knowledge is the discovery of something we do not understand." Frank Herbert

I have told you about a few of the strange events which took place shortly after Madeleine's departure from this world. Those after-death communication events gave me a sense of comfort and helped me enormously in trying to find answers about life and death. I started questioning people from different faiths and cultures about their beliefs. I could not believe how common these after-death communication events were. In fact, my enquiry seemed to provide people with an outlet to talk about their own personal after-death communication experience with their loved ones. They poured their hearts out. Together with their stories, my own experiences and through my personal research into after-death communication I was beginning to believe that Madeleine was indeed communicating with me. The reactions that I had from people when I answered their questions as to how I was faring ranged from one of disbelief and dismissal to *'tell me more about these after-death communication events'*.

If I had been told about after-death communication events prior to my own personal experience, I would have expressed an 'open but unconvinced' opinion about same.

Some people however, were very harsh and issued me with advice to remove and or dispose of all things that reminded me of Madeleine. *"It is time for you to move on and live your life"* they said. That attitude shocked me. What most people didn't realise was the fact that my love for Madeleine had never been stronger and even now, I love her more than ever. The love that we had for each other on earth seems to have attained a spiritual dimension far deeper than any love we shared before.

Within me there is a strange peace which I can only put down to some sort of spiritual enlightenment. Interestingly, those people telling me to move on and break away from Madeleine, have all had disastrous relationships. As I am writing this book, almost one year on from Madeleine's departure from this earthly world, Madeleine's things at home are still in their usual places. I will only start giving her things away when my heart tells me it is time to do so. People may think that I am going crazy but as far as I am concerned, Madeleine is still around in a spiritual sense and I find great comfort talking to her all the time.

Whether a believer, a cynic or still sitting on the fence as regards after-death communication, you are entitled to your opinion and it is not my intention to persuade you to think any differently. What I would like to do however is share some of my personal experience on after-death communication events and let you see how they are helping me to come to terms with the devastating loss of my wife and have brought me to a point in my life that has given me a new hope and a reason to live again.

Friday April 8, 2011. I had been feeling really down, very sad and desperately lonely. Little things that reminded me of Madeleine made me worse. The tears were almost non-stop as I was missing her so much. On several occasions, I had been asking her to give me courage to carry on. After dinner, I cleaned up the dishes and brought in the laundry. Then, I went into the bedroom to put things away in the walk-in wardrobe. When I entered the bedroom, I noticed that there was a deep head imprint on my top pillow which had also been moved into an angled position. Madeleine always tidied the bed in the morning and fluffed the pillows leaving no head imprints. She was very meticulous in this routine and you may remember me telling you earlier that I had continued this routine so as not to make it appear only half the bed was used. The doona cover and top bed sheet had also been moved away from the pillow.

That same night, whilst I was tidying up the kitchen I noticed something else unusual. The formal dining room is only used when we have guests or have more than four people dining. Annabelle and I had eaten dinner at the kitchen bench extension so no one had been into the dining room. The dining table and chairs were kept meticulously tidy the way Madeleine liked it, with all the chairs always tucked under the table. Much to my surprise, the chair where Madeleine normally sat had been moved backwards as if someone had been sitting on this chair at the table. How do you explain this? I could think of no logical explanation.

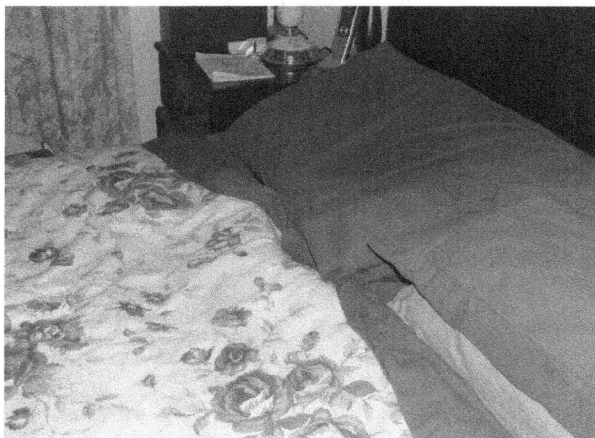

The strange pillow indent

Monday April 11, 2011. Flying back on a Virgin Blue flight from Sydney to Melbourne, I was half asleep and was suddenly woken by the sight of Madeleine looking at me.

She was very real, not dream like at all. It was definitely Madeleine looking at me with her usual smile.

Saturday April 16, 2011. Annabelle was suffering from continual abdominal pain, a condition she has had on and off for years. The pain was so severe she had to be taken to the Dandenong Private Hospital. On the way to hospital, I was seeking Madeleine's help to look after Annabelle and asking her to make sure that Annabelle was OK. Annabelle was admitted to the emergency ward and her boyfriend Miguel and I were waiting for the results of the ultrasound scans and X-ray. I may have dozed off but was suddenly aware of Madeleine and Annabelle side by side looking at me, in a bright and blue sky environment. I jumped up and startled both Annabelle and Miguel. A few minutes later, the doctor came in with the results and told Annabelle that she was suffering a minor treatable bowel condition. A reason had at last been found for this recurrent abdominal pain which for years had baffled doctors. Could this have been Madeleine's doing?

Saturday April 23, 2011. Whilst lying in bed, I felt a very strong presence as if Madeleine was on the other side of the bed. I even turned around to reach for her but she was not there. Nevertheless, I spoke to her and asked her to let me know that she was OK.

This was not the first time I had held what I can only describe as an amazing in-depth conversation with Madeleine. With not a single word or sound exchanged, the intensity of thought did the talking. Invariably the response was the same, a strong feeling that she was always there, listening.

Sunday April 24, 2011. I had dinner at our elder son Gerard's place and returned home rather late. I wanted to work on the May edition of the Mauritius Australia Connection Newsletter before retiring for the night. At 11.30 pm I was sitting at my desk typing away when I felt a gentle but firm tug on the left hand sleeve of my T shirt. I turned just in time to observe my left hand sleeve being pinched and pulled back some 2-3 cms. I was shocked and remained motionless for some minutes.

I said nothing about this to nobody until two weeks later. Annabelle and I were having dinner and I walked up behind her, pinched and pulled back the left hand sleeve of her T shirt the same way as mine had been pulled that night. She looked at me and said: *"Why are you doing this to me, only Meme (Madeleine) does this."* I told her what had happened to me. This pinching of the left hand sleeve was a habit of Madeleine's used only with Annabelle and me.

She was left handed and would elegantly pinch your left hand sleeve with her left hand to get your attention.

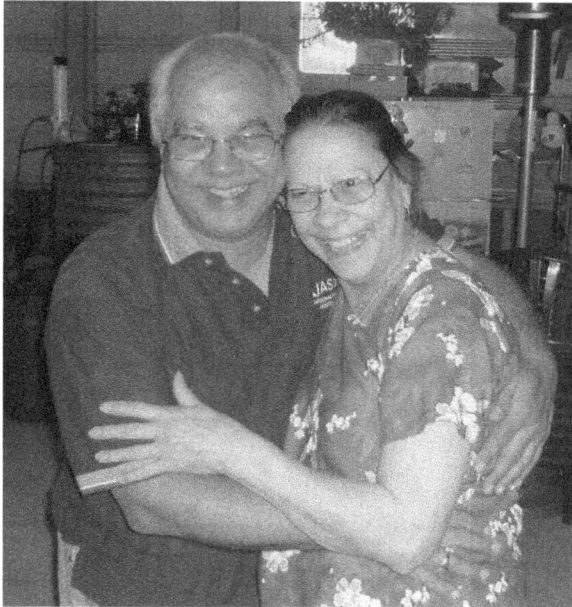

Clancy wearing the T-Shirt that Madeleine tugged

Annabelle's reaction confirmed what I had suspected, that the tug on my sleeve two weeks previously was indeed Madeleine sending me a signal and letting me know that she was "still alive and in good spirits". I can think of no other possible explanation.

Sunday May 15, 2011. When visiting Madeleine at the Springvale Botanical Cemetery, I said to her that it had been a while since she had come to see me. That night, at 3.15 am, I awoke and felt someone gently stroking the doona cover. I sat up, checked the doona cover and tried to fall asleep again. I felt the same stroking movements again. It had to be Madeleine.

Friday May 27, 2011. I kissed Madeleine's photo goodnight and told her about people telling me to get on with my life and not to think too much about her. I assured her this was not going to happen and she was not to worry about it. In the very early hours of the morning, around 12.39 am, I felt something strange was happening on the left hand side of the bed. Someone was repeatedly touching the doona cover.

I opened my eyes to see a body shaped pulsating viscous air column between the ceiling and the bed. I blinked several times thinking that I was imagining it but the same viscous air column - v shaped at the bottom and widened to some 30 cms at the top – was still there. The pulsating lasted for about 2-3 minutes with the soft touch on the doona cover continuing as well. Then everything stopped and the viscous air column cleared.

Friday June 10, 2011. I was watching a DVD and fell asleep in the same armchair that Madeleine used to occupy. I woke up to see Madeleine, dressed in one of her long kaftan robes, looking at me with an expression of concern, as if she was asking me to be careful.

Monday June 13, 2011. I was in bed and awakened by the feeling that Madeleine was in front of me, cuddling me with open arms. I was immediately overcome with this incredible reality that she was in the bedroom watching over me.

This made me very happy and very sad at the same time. Whether half dream/half reality or not, it was a most overwhelming feeling that just cannot be explained. Until you experience such an event, you just would not comprehend this overwhelming sensation.

Saturday June 25, 2011. I was invited to dinner with some friends of ours. Madeleine's brother Jean was also there. He told me that he had this most unusual dream of Madeleine and their mother Thérèse. The latter told Jean in his dream not to worry, that Madeleine was with her and that she was OK and in her care.

Thursday June 30, 2011. I had a shower before going to bed at my usual time of 10.30 pm. That night, I had been in and out of the bedroom twice before going into the bathroom - everything was looking normal. When I came out of the bathroom to get into bed, I noticed that the top pillow had moved into a 45 degree angle against the lower pillow, and had a head print on it, similar to the one that appeared a few months earlier. This time I examined the pillow more closely. The head print was too small to be mine and was definitely more the size of Madeleine's head. I was alone in the house and besides, nobody ever goes into my bedroom.

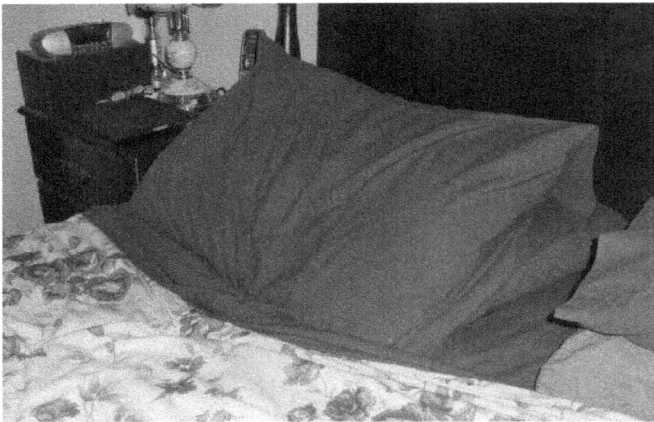

Another strange pillow indent

That head print on the pillow appeared from nowhere and can only be explained by some extraordinary event. I was more convinced than ever that Madeleine must again have paid me a visit.

On every occasion that Madeleine manifested her presence, I would have been very down, crying and missing her so much that it was really hurting.

Her presence almost invariably boosted my spirit and eased my sadness. Annabelle suggested that we consult a medium. We both went to the Lyceum Childs Spiritual Church in Brunswick, Melbourne.

Annabelle and I met with the medium separately and she had no idea that we were related. It was just amazing how much she knew of Madeleine. For example, she told Annabelle that the watch that she was wearing belonged to someone else and carried a lot of love with it. The watch belonged to Madeleine and I gave it to Annabelle after Madeleine passed away. The medium told me that she could see Madeleine with a little dog (her description fitted Kimby, a little Jack Russell terrier that we had for years). She also told me that Madeleine was very happy with the way that Annabelle had progressed in her career. The most incredible thing that the medium told me was that I would be receiving signs of Madeleine's presence.

She also told me that I would be going on holidays in three months' time. (I had just booked a trip to Mauritius and Europe in October only the week before).

Following the visit to the medium, and throughout the month of July, Madeleine was leaving signs of her presence on a regular basis: pillow head prints, ruffled bed sheets and folded back doona covers on her side of the bed and on one occasion I even felt that my feet were being pulled down into a straight position. Every time these unexplained events happened, I could not help but cry for joy that Madeleine was still very much with me.

Wednesday July 27, 2011. Gerard and the boys were at my place and we were talking about Madeleine. Gerard was telling me that only a few days before Madeleine died, she told him how worried she was about what would happen to me. The previous day, I had taken Madeleine's signet ring from her jewellery box as she had always told Gerard that the ring would be his when she died.

I went into the bedroom to get it and immediately noticed the top pillow had moved again into its now customary angled position, with the indented head print there for all to see. I called Gerard in to show him. He burst into tears and we both became very emotional.

On August 3, 9, 16 and 26, 2011, similar movements of the top pillow with the head indent within were observed. Interestingly, whenever this happened I went to bed and placed my head exactly into the indent. Every single time, I fell straight into deep sleep mode.

Around the same time, I received a reply to an email I had sent to Dr Michael Barbaro, specialist in palliative care and after-death communication research.

I had told him about the experiences I had been having prior to and since Madeleine's death.

He writes:

"Hi Clancy

Thank you for the email and details concerning your experiences before and after Madeleine's death.

It's hard to know where to start. The most important thing to appreciate is that the experiences you have described following Madeleine's death are very common and very normal. Why they arise and what they mean is controversial and is a debate I prefer to avoid simply because reason and logic are incapable of grasping the mystery of death. In instances such as you have described we believe what we believe because of the effect the experience has upon us.

The experience may not make sense but it feels real, often more real than other 'earthly' events. These are precious gifts.

Many people will question or doubt the things you have described or they may dismiss them saying, 'your mind is playing tricks'. Never doubt the truth or the significance of the experiences, be grateful for them and ask, 'what is Madeleine trying to tell me'?

I hope that these words are of help. Happy to elaborate further if necessary. My website may also be helpful
www.caringforthedying.com.au

Best wishes
Michael"

Sunday October 2, 2011. I took time off from writing this book as it was too painful for me to keep going. I had to have a box of tissues beside me as I was crying all the time when I was writing. The pain eased off a bit, except that simple things triggered the memory bank and I could not help recall some of the great times that Madeleine and I spent together. Invariably, the tears flowed as a result of this. That Sunday, I spent the afternoon cooking one of Madeleine's favourite dishes. Whilst I was cooking, I conversed with her as if she was present in the kitchen. Needless to say, I was crying all the time. I went to bed feeling really sad and spent a fair bit of time looking at photos of Madeleine on my iPad through the tears. My mood could not have been lower.

When I pulled the doona cover over me and switched off the bedside lamp, I could feel very noticeable caressing movements on the doona cover from the upper legs to the shoulder. I stopped breathing to see if it was my breathing that was causing these movements.

I even got out of bed to check if the air conditioning was somehow causing this to happen. The air conditioning was off and the air in the bedroom was still. I went back to bed and covered myself. I could feel the same caress/stroking movements on the doona and immediately burst into tears as I realised this could only be Madeleine. Knowing how very sad I was, she had come to comfort me.

The day before I had been suffering from unusual body pains and could not walk properly without winching. Madeleine used to have similar joint pains and I remember at the time thinking that it was probably my turn to have some sort of arthritis. Miraculously, when I woke up the next morning, all pain had disappeared. For some strange reason, this reminded me that Madeleine would also suffer from foot cramps, with so much pain that she had to get up and put weight on her feet to stop the pain. Immediately I reflected on the previous night's events and remembered that when I had felt the stroking movement over the doona cover during the night, I was also feeling these same foot cramps. Was Madeleine trying to tell me something?

Up until now, the visits from Madeleine had more often than not, been when I was on familiar ground and grieving.

From the tiniest of revelations and the visions of her presence to feeling her touch and sensing her perfume, all were given exactly the same importance in my heart.

Sunday October 9, 2011. I received an email from Monique and François Catta owners of *'Chateau des Rangeardieres'* in Saint Barthélemy nears Angers in France, inviting me to stay with them at the chateau during my European vacations.

Monique and François Catta are respectively Countess de St Exupery and Count Catta in their own rights. This chateau was owned by Madeleine's ancestors from 1807 to 1819. The family then included Claude Valentin Paruit d'Esmery, his wife Agathe, daughter Valentine and the two sons Auguste and Henry.

Claude Paruit d'Esmery was a very high profile figure both before and during the Napoleonic era. In fact, Claude and his two sons fought in the *'Grande Armée'* during the Russian campaign and the Battle of Waterloo. Auguste and Henry were boy soldiers. Claude and Henry are direct ancestors of Madeleine.

Madeleine and I spent considerable time tracking back our family trees. I cried realizing that she was not going to be with me during the visit.

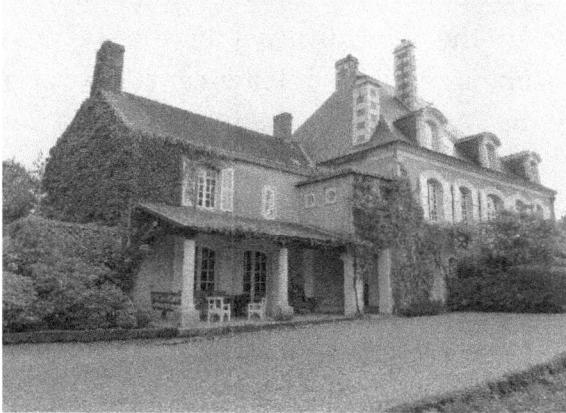

The Paruit's ancestral home 'Chateau des Rangeardieres'

However, in my own way I spoke to Madeleine and said to her: *"You'd better be there when I shall be at the 'Chateau des Rangeardieres'."*

The spiritual bond between us was growing stronger by the day. Little did I know that I was about to discover my after-death communication with Madeleine was soon to take on a whole new meaning and we were about to head back to Europe.

Tuesday October 25, 2011, I was on the 11.15 am TGV (Train à Grande Vitesse) 8913 leaving Gare de Montparnasse in Paris for Angers.

François Catta would be waiting for me in Angers to take me to the *'Chateau des Rangeardieres'* in Saint Barthélemy. I was seated in the window seat of the TGV. A lady of about the same age as Madeleine came and occupied the seat beside me. We started our journey. I was minding my own business when the lady struck up a conversation by telling me that she was going to Angers to meet with friends. I told her that I was from Melbourne, Australia and was also going to Angers. She then said to me *"You are meeting with friends too."* I responded in the affirmative.

At some point in time, she told me that she was going to the buffet carriage for something to eat. She left and some fifteen minutes later, I left to go to the buffet carriage as well.

I could not see her there and spent some twenty minutes having a drink and a sandwich. I returned to my seat. The lady had not yet returned to hers. She came back some fifteen minutes later and told me that she was looking for me. I found this a bit strange and did not pay any attention to her remark.

A short time later, she bent over to pick up a folded crosswords magazine in her bag which was lying on the floor in front of her.

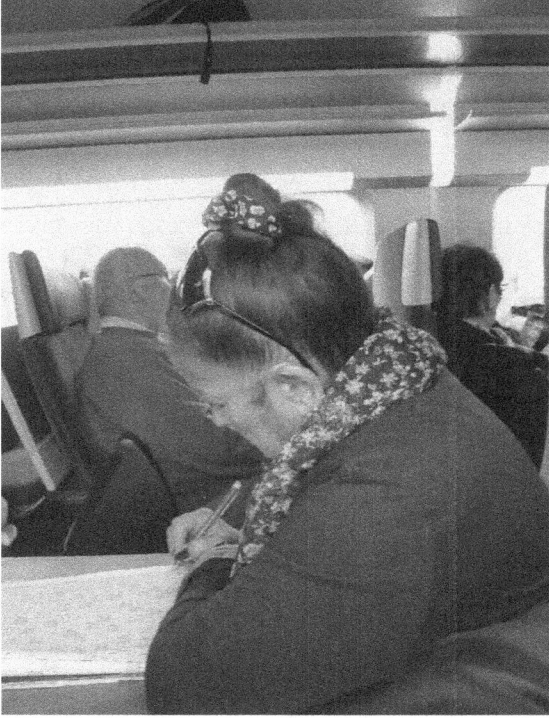

Travel Companion on the train to Angers

The magazine looked very much the same as the one to which Madeleine subscribed in Melbourne. She got her pen out from the folded magazine, very much the same way that Madeleine kept her pen. She was doing the crosswords and I could not help thinking that *'it was almost as if Madeleine was there beside me'*. Then, I had the shock of my life.

The lady turned to me and asked: *"Marsupial from Australia, you should know this."* I was stunned and speechless and before I could answer, she said: *"Koala."*

Madeleine, just before she became very ill, enjoyed doing crosswords in bed. I remember very clearly one night when we were in bed she asked me: *"Marsupial from Australia, you should know this"* and before I could answer, she said: *"Koala."* Exactly the same way as the lady on the train had done. I was speechless and then it struck me like a ton of bricks - only a fortnight ago I had asked Madeleine to come with me when I visited the *'Chateau des Rangeardieres'*. Madeleine was keeping her side of the bargain. In her own way, she had accompanied me on my way to Angers. How do you explain this?

I took a photo of the lady in a discrete manner without her noticing. I was watching her and could not help observing that her fingernails had red nail varnish similar to Madeleine's.

Her hair was done up in the same casual 'tucked pony tail' manner that Madeleine sometimes used.

From the photo, I later realized that her greyish black and white overcoat was very much in the same style as a similar overcoat that Madeleine had - refer to the photo at the start of Chapter 8. People to whom I have shown the photo have told me that if I superimposed Madeleine's face profile into the photo, they would swear that it was Madeleine.

There was more to come, the train conductor announced that we were to arrive at St Laud train station in Angers within the next twenty minutes. The lady folded up her crosswords magazine, tucked the pen in and pushed it into her bag, in very much the same way as Madeleine would. She then grabbed hold of a red lipstick from her bag and proceeded to put lipstick on her lips just like Madeleine would. I was lost for words. How do you explain this 'synchronicity' of events that very much recreated Madeleine's presence on the seat next to me in the same train that was taking me to Angers.

Incidentally, during my stay at *'Chateau des Rangeardieres'* I took many photographs including the garden landscape on the front cover. The garden itself was conceived and built by Madeleine's ancestor Claude Valentin Paruit d'Esmery who owned the property from 1809 – 1819.

This garden represents a real connection between the past and present. On my return to Melbourne, I had a closer look at that photo and could not explain the presence of a unique 'purple haze' covering the walkway. It certainly was not visible to the naked eye when I took the shot nor did it appear in any of the other photos taken at the same time. Some people to whom I had shown the photo, told me that this purple haze had a special significance. This had to be Madeleine's way of responding to my conversations with her, in particular my demand that she had better be at *'Chateau des Rangeardieres'*.

More recently, a good friend of mine undertook the editing of the manuscript for this book. One night we communicated over the internet for more than an hour and edited the book manuscript as we went along. When I was closing down the multiple 'Internet Explorer' tabs on my desktop, the monitor screen lit up with multiple fluorescent 'purple patches' flashing on the tabs. The shade of purple was identical to the 'purple haze' that infiltrated the garden landscape photo.

A short time after the internet conversation, I had cause to look at the photo of my 'travel companion' to Angers, and could not believe my eyes when I noticed that the train seats' upholstery, the lady's hair clip, some of the motifs on her collar and even her pen were all purple.

Surely all this could no longer be classed as coincidence: the synchronicity of Madeleine's earlier visits; the seemingly incarnate presence on the train; the appearance of a purple hue in several very different scenarios and the strong feeling that Madeleine was with me throughout the visit at *'Chateau des Rangeardieres'*.

Together these events had to be the solid evidence that my engineering mind had been so eagerly seeking as proof that after-death communication did occur. There definitely were higher forces at work.

Chapter 14

Touch of an Angel

"If I could reach up and hold a star for every time you've made me smile, the entire evening sky would be in the palm of my hand." – Anon

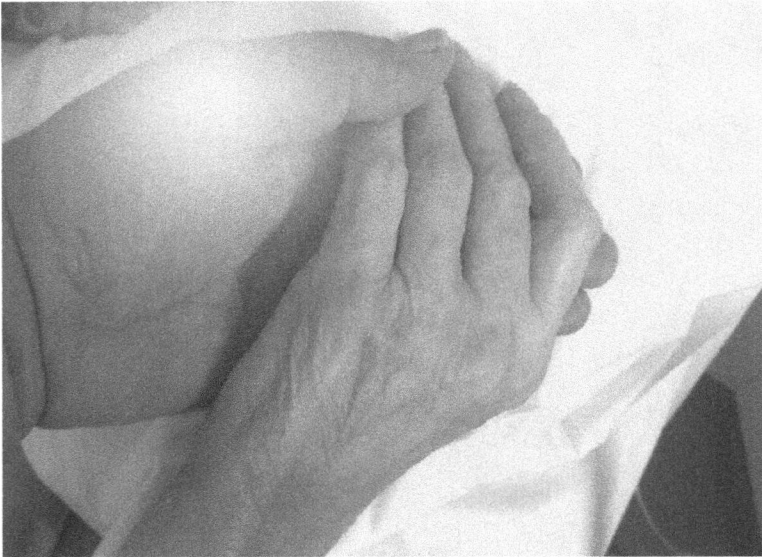

Madeleine and Clancy holding hands

One night in the midst of grief, I could not help but see Madeleine's beautiful hands in front of me.

Words came rushing out from deep within my soul and this is what my heart wrote.

Your hands were the most loving that could be

In times of need, the touch of your hands brought comfort and peace. I feel the absence of your hands because the good things in life do not last forever.

Your hands carried so much love that I have cause to believe that your hands will always be around to care for me.

The magic touch of your hands filled my heart with joy and ensured that we were but one self, bonded to each other. When I was hungry, your hands methodically and lovingly prepared delicious foods that we would enjoy and share with others around the world.

I have seen your hands comfort the down and out and give them reason to carry on with hope and trust in God. Your hands brought me to reason when I lost my way and started to wander.

Your hands tilled the soil, dug up the weeds and sowed the seeds that would bring the flowers to welcome the change in seasons. My efforts in home improvements and other things would have amounted to nothing if your loving hands were not there to help me and give me courage to carry on.

I always looked well cared for because your hands made sure that the clothes I wore were the very best.

When we walked around, your hands proudly held on to mine, to publicly proclaim our undying love for each other. The touch of your hands was enough to symbolise the unconditional love that we had for each other. Words were not necessary as your hands spoke their own language of love.

Your hands endured the trauma of chemotherapy, never giving up and always on the ready for the next challenge. In the middle of the night, your hands touched me and caressed me to sleep so that tomorrow was something worth waking up to.

When I was hurting or felt unwell, your hands would be there offering comfort and solace in remedies that only loved ones can provide.

You wore our wedding and engagement rings on your hands proudly displayed to show the world that we were bonded for life and in the thereafter.

Your hands held on to mine with so much love, in spite of the hard times you went through that I can still feel your loving touch to this day.

The day the Lord took you into his care, the touch of your hands stayed with me.

I have no doubt that your hands are still caring for me in more ways than I can imagine. Your unique left hand tug came to me to let me know that you were OK.

Your loving hands will always be with me because they are very much part of me now. The touch of an angel that will always be part of my life, now and thereafter.

Chapter 15

When do the Tears Stop?

"Some people come into our lives and quickly go. Some people move our souls to dance. They awaken us to a new understanding with the passing whisper of their wisdom. Some people make the sky more beautiful to gaze upon. They stay in our lives for awhile, leave footprints on our hearts, and we are never, ever the same." Flavia Weedn

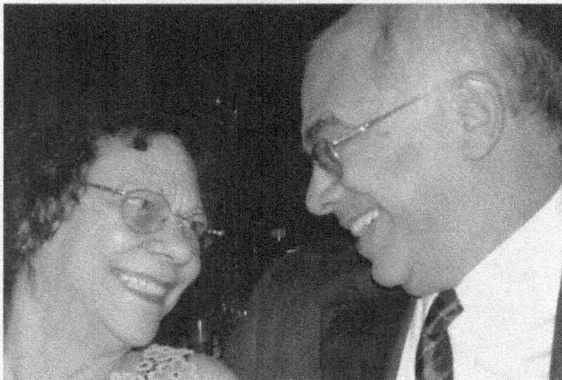

Madeleine and Clancy 'Eyes doing the talking'

Immediately after Madeleine's death, I felt that life was not worth living and objectively felt that I would not recover from this fatal blow.

My engineering background told me there was no possible solution on this earth which could lead to a recovery and enable me to get on with the rest of my life without Madeleine. The bottom had dropped out of my world. Madeleine meant everything to me. I lived for her and her for me. She was not there anymore.

Where was I to go from that point? There had been no grief and pain to compare with the absolute loss I felt with the death of my soul mate, wife, best friend and confidante. The unconditional love that Madeleine had for me was gone and that drove me to despair. I seriously understood why people in similar situations contemplated suicide. I did too, but discounted this as the easy way out. This would cause even more pain to the loved ones that I would leave behind.

The least little thing would suddenly trigger the pain and bring the tears streaming down my face. Little things like the memory of her laughter and the way she did things that now I had to do for myself in her absence had me crying nearly every single day.

The grief, frightening at times left me desolated in my emotions. I was on the downslide and things could only get worse. I was finished and heading for depression.

My loved ones offered the best support they could, encouraging me by saying that time would heal the pain and grief.

My own doctor virtually insisted on prescribing antidepressants and sleeping pills. I categorically refused this option and remarked that that was not a solution at all.

However, it was the paranormal events that occurred subsequent to Madeleine's death which suddenly provided a glimpse of hope and a much needed light at the end of the tunnel. As my engineering expertise had failed miserably to find logical explanations for these events, my thinking was forced to diversify into the realms of the impossible becoming possible and to accept that there were indeed things that could not be physically explained within the limitations of our comprehension of things. The paranormal events that I witnessed after Madeleine's death had provided the solid proof I was seeking.

My extensive research into the subject of after-death communication and finding out that other people had undergone similar experiences helped to convince me, (and hopefully others) that I was not heading for cuckoo land.

I am reminded of the contents of an email sent to me by Dr Michael Barbato which proved to be a major turning point in my thinking:

"The most important thing to appreciate is that the experiences you have described following Madeleine's death are very common and very normal.

Why they arise and what they mean is controversial and is a debate I prefer to avoid simply because reason and logic are incapable of grasping the mystery of death. In instances such as you have described we believe what we believe because of the effect the experience has upon us. The experience may not make sense but it feels real, often more real than other 'earthly' events. These are precious gifts."

I am now totally convinced that these events were after-death communications from Madeleine. Whilst her body, ravaged by the impact of the breast and ovarian cancers, had died, her 'spiritual being' had survived. I was much comforted by the realisation that Madeleine's 'spiritual being' was communicating with me and letting me know that she was not totally gone. From then on, the downward slide seemed to go into reverse and I began to feel so much better, my whole outlook changed and I started to move forward. I had come to accept that Madeleine was better off where she was as all physical pain had gone, and in my heart I knew that sometime in the future, we would be together reunited again.

I had learnt that even in death there can be comfort, that my love for Madeleine cannot and will never die; that communication with her could still go on. I had found new ways of loving. Out of pain, grief and deep sadness came an awareness of Madeleine's spiritual presence that was very real.

This higher awareness of life and death caused very profound changes in my beliefs, trust in God, love for people and a very marked shift in my attachment to material things. I have placed a much higher importance on love for my close family and on having greater consideration for others.

Come to think of it, this was Madeleine's simple yet religious approach to life. For years I had admired this philosophy of hers and accepted it was something that Madeleine always did. With this shift in my own focus on life has come the realization that I am in fact living life the way Madeleine herself would have done.

Is it possible that there are deeper forces at work in my life? Shortly after Madeleine's death, I felt an incredible emptiness believing a huge part of me had died too.

With everything that has happened since her passing I am reminded that there is an even bigger part of Madeleine still living in my life.

Madeleine and I had been soul mates all our lives, and there seems to be more and more evidence gathering to prove not even death can tear us apart.

The following extract was taken from *'Soul Mates, Spiritual Happiness and Family Love'* section on *'Soul Mates, Marriage in Heaven'* at http://www.cjp.net

"We were spiritually married and continue that relationship into eternity. Couples united like this in marriage think and breathe permanence, and their eternal happiness is based on this idea. For all these reasons they are no longer two but one person - that is, one flesh. To spiritual eyes it is plainly clear that they cannot be torn apart by either one's death.

That these two are not even separated by the death of one, since the spirit of the deceased husband or wife continues to live with the wife or husband who is not yet deceased. And this continues until the other one's death, when they meet again and reunite themselves and love each other more tenderly than before because they are in the spiritual world."

This change in my own thinking has intensified my deep love for Madeleine already.

Together, with the wonderful support of the loved ones, I have become emotionally and indeed spiritually stronger than I have ever been before.

Amazing things continue to happen. Madeleine and I were very passionate about Mauritian Cuisine. We would talk at length about the preparation of Mauritian dishes and other dishes for that matter. Many hours were spent with me taking notes and measuring the quantities of ingredients that Madeleine would use in her cooking for different dishes.

Madeleine had the knack of cooking by instinct and she would also assess the progression of her cooking for everything that she cooked with surgical precision. She would adjust the incorporation of ingredients and flavours by adding a bit of this and a bit of that, to get the right balance. I followed through by taking notes, writing up the recipes and elaborating on the cooking steps with engineering precision. The combination of her culinary skills and my engineering background resulted in recipes that were virtually fail proof.

After Madeleine died, I had no other option but to cook for myself when our elder son Gerard was not staying at home with me. Initially, I had to keep referring to Madeleine's notes and the numerous recipes that we had put together.

Out of the blue, and much to my surprise, I suddenly found myself cooking in exactly the same way as Madeleine did.

As if by magic I was instinctively preparing Madeleine's dishes and feeling that Madeleine was in the kitchen behind me guiding my hands to make sure that I did the right thing. These days, cooking Madeleine's favourite dishes is like therapy for me. It creates some sort of spiritual connection between us. Whilst I am cooking, I find myself talking to her all the time and occasionally when I am lost in terms of what to do next, I ask myself the question *"What would Madeleine have done?"*

Almost immediately, the answer comes to me. This deep 'thought talking' has become something very special on my road to recovery and has helped me enormously to see the smiles through the tears.

In March 2012, I had positive results from a preliminary test for bowel cancer. My doctor advised that I took further tests and underwent an endoscopy.

I was revisiting the waiting game that we had when Madeleine undertook her cancer tests. For some strange reason, I was calm and did not have any trouble at all accepting the fact that if the endoscopy showed signs of bowel cancer, I could also be facing a battle with cancer too.

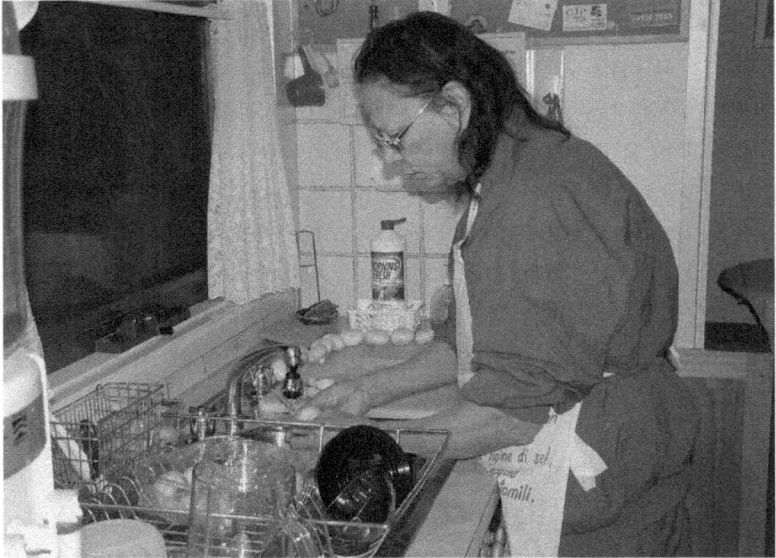

Madeleine is always present in the background

I was not scared of dying. In fact, I felt comfortable with crossing the 'divide' to rejoin my beloved Madeleine. As it turned out, the endoscopy results were negative and I was OK. However, I felt very emotional after the procedure and visited Madeleine at the cemetery. I cried as I told her the results that the endoscopy indicated benign cysts which had been removed and no malignancy found.

Upon my return home, I entered my bedroom to see that there was an indent in my top pillow. Madeleine had paid me a visit to let me know that she received the good news. This is real *'Eternal Love for each other.'*

My connection with the family has become stronger than ever and every single day Madeleine's influence protects and guides us all. This little episode illustrates perfectly that Madeleine is still very much present among us. I was driving my grandsons Brandon and Joshua around and was not really concentrating on my driving which to say the least was erratic.

Brandon and Joshua told their Dad Gerard that they had to talk to him about something very important. Dad kept avoiding the issue until one night after dinner the boys insisted that Dad listen. They told him that they were concerned about my driving.

"It is getting dangerous," they said. They had to keep telling me to apply the brakes or stop as I was an accident waiting to happen. Dad responded *"It was Ok because you were both with him and nothing happened."* They queried: *"What would happen when he is driving the car alone by himself?"* Dad responded: *"Don't worry Meme (Madeleine) is with him all the time."* The two boys said: *"That's OK then."*

I have had some interesting observations from people. One friend after realising that I was still very much in love with Madeleine said: *"I never thought that people could love like that."* To many, this might seem incongruous and irrational. The fact is that I do feel that the love between us is still very real and more intense. Whilst Madeleine may not be here in bodily form, her spiritual presence is very much with me all the time.

Two Mauritian Community radio programs broadcasting in Melbourne, Australia and Brighton on Hove in the United Kingdom, paid tribute to this unconditional love that I have for Madeleine. Their choices of fitting songs to accompany one radio interview and an announcement about Madeleine and myself were *'Aimer jusqu'a l'impossible'* (Love to the impossible) by Tina Arena and *'Je t'aimais, je t'aime et je t'aimerai'* (I loved you, still love you and will always love you) by Francis Cabrel.

I feel now that I am a man on a mission. My mission is to complete the unfinished tasks that Madeleine and I set off on our journey together to do. I need to finish this book and put on record the caring, loving and wonderful person that Madeleine was. In particular, to pass on to future generations the loving memories of their ancestral grandmother and how bravely she fought through her five year battle with breast and ovarian cancers.

We were also very intent on recording in a book, Madeleine's concept of Mauritian Cuisine. In particular, Madeleine's appreciation of Mauritian Cuisine the way it should be. I will of course continue to maintain the world famous *'Mauritius Australia Connection'* web site, incorporating the equally and very popular world famous *'Recipes from Mauritius'* web site.

The continuing tributes to Madeleine coming from her friends worldwide are also testament to the huge support that I am still getting through emails and postings.

A great supporter of Madeleine's recipes over the years has been Henri Maurel, a Mauritian living in Southern France. Henri created a special dish in Madeleine's memory named *'Saumon Maddy-Saveur des Iles'*. I was extremely touched by this. Furthermore, Henri has translated many of Madeleine's recipes into French thus allowing a wider audience access to her menus.

Madeleine is still very much alive, criss-crossing the stars through the world wide web network and bringing the comfort of her popular dishes into the homes of millions. Today, I am enjoying the presence and love of my nearest and dearest and looking forward to the day when I will be reunited with my beloved Madeleine. Meanwhile, she lives on within us through the good memories, the

children, the grandchildren and the great granddaughter
Lilly Madeleine.

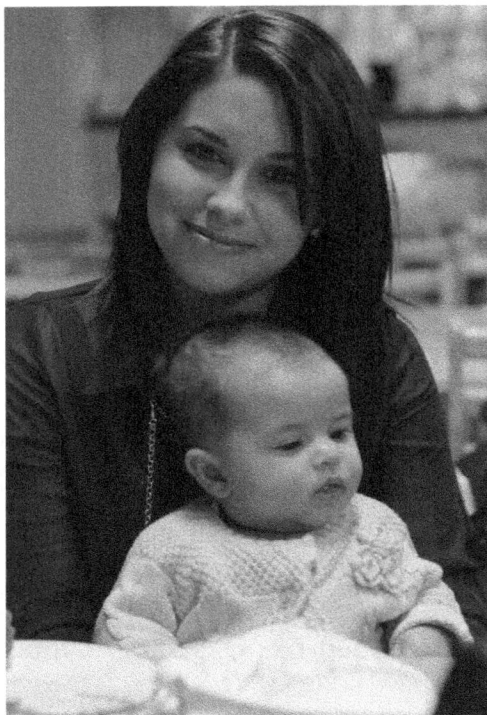

Annabelle and Lilly Madeleine

I have an added bonus in that I am now a great
grandfather. Annabelle gave birth on April 5, 2012 to a
daughter named Lilly Madeleine and is already showing
signs of being a wonderful mother just as Madeleine was.

The naming of the daughter after Madeleine was a blessing for me.

When I look at mother and daughter, many of Madeleine's attributes are already apparent. The other grandchildren also carry much of Madeleine's personality in them.

When do the tears stop? Well, I do not think that the tears will ever stop for me. Madeleine has been too much a part of my life for me not to shed tears when the memories of the good times we had together come flashing through my mind.

The only thing is that time and the comfort of her 'spiritual presence' have made my recovery from the tears much, much easier. Every now and then the pain of grief still grabs me and the tears come rolling down my cheeks like a tap in full flow. After a while, I am OK and get back to living life with Madeleine still very much part of it.

The truth is that I am more in love with Madeleine now than I have ever been before. You learn to love in different ways. Since her passing, the memories we shared are very much alive, especially the loving moments that we spent together.

It is as if our love has blossomed in a new enlightened dimension where we can once again enjoy times together and find new ways of giving and receiving love through this 'spiritual presence'.

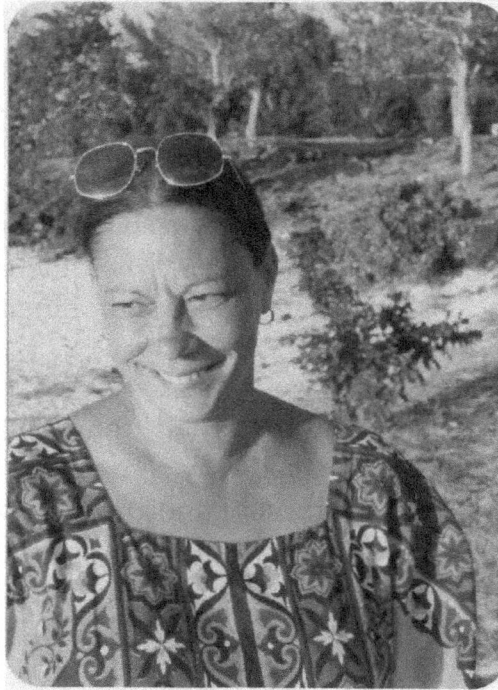

Madeleine as I saw her in my after-death vision

I hope that our experience becomes a beacon of light for others in their journeys through grief or tragedy.

"What greater thing is there for two human souls than to feel that they are joined together to strengthen each other in all labour, to minister to each other in all sorrow, to share with each other in all gladness, to be one with each other in the silent unspoken memories." George Eliot

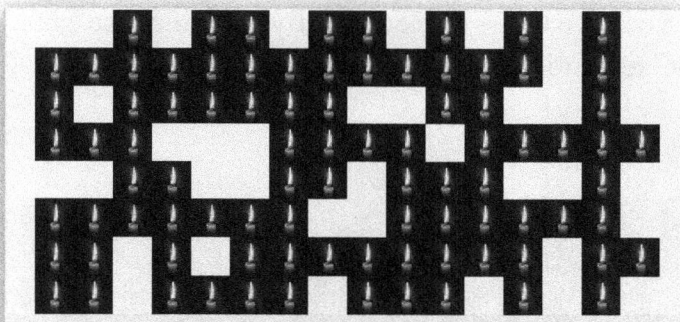

You can light a candle on Madeleine's Memorial web site at: **http://www.ilasting.com/madeleinephilippe.php**

Chapter 16

'Til we meet again....

"And if I could live my life all over again, it would still be with you. No one else can offer you a heart so true. No one else can love you like I do." Anon

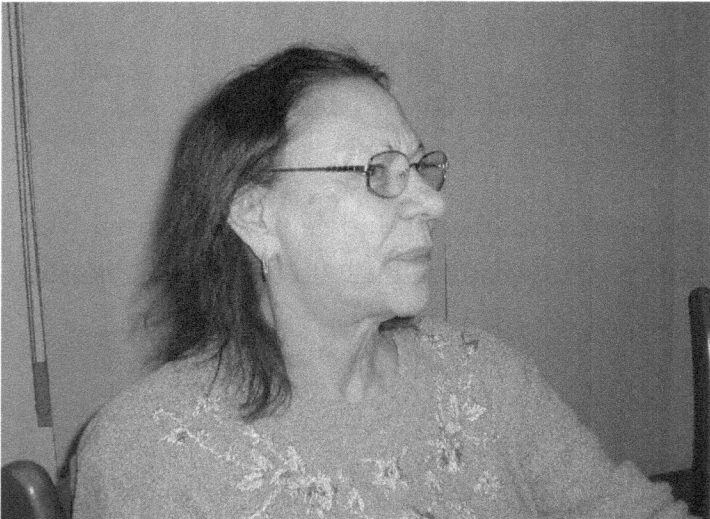

'I will always love you'

"I'm well, I'm fine, I'm here"

I stood by your bed last night.
I came to have a peep.
I could see that you were crying,
You found it hard to sleep.

I touched you softly as you brushed away a tear,
'It's me, I haven't left you, I'm well, I'm fine, I'm here.'

I was close to you at breakfast,
I watched you pour the coffee.
You were thinking of the many times

Your hands reached down to me.
I gently put my hand on you, I smiled and said 'It's me.'

You looked so very tired as you sank into the sofa.
I tried so hard to let you know I was standing there.

It's possible for me to be so near you every day,
To say with certainty, 'I never went away.'
You sat there quietly, then smiled, I think you knew.
In the stillness of that evening, I was very close to you.

The day is over....
I smile and watch you yawning and say
'Good night, God bless, I'll see you in the morning.'

And when the time is right for you to cross the brief divide,
I'll rush across to greet you and we'll stand side by side.
I have so many things to show you,
There is so much for you to see.

Be patient, live your journey out...then come to be with me.

Author unknown

Madeleine Philippe Cancer Foundation

Madeleine Philippe Cancer Foundation (Aus) Inc
http://www.mpcfaus.org

"So that we may help others and save lives, through raising breast and ovarian cancer awareness through sharing knowledge and experience."

The proceeds from the publication of this book will be donated to the Foundation.

Additional support is always appreciated. You can donate directly via the donation link on the foundation's web site. All proceeds will be spent in the promotion of breast and ovarian cancer awareness and their early detection.

The Madeleine Philippe Cancer Foundation (Aus) Inc is registered as a non profit charitable organisation in the State of Victoria, Australia. Registration No. A0052688B under the Associations Incorporation Act 1981. State of Victoria in Australia. Rules of the Foundation are available upon request.

Join the foundation support group on Facebook:
http://www.facebook.com/groups/mpcfaus/

About the Author

Clancy Philippe, born in Mauritius, graduated at the City University in London in 1970, with a Honours Degree in Civil Engineering. He has since pursued a professional career in Local Government in the United Kingdom, Mauritius and Australia.

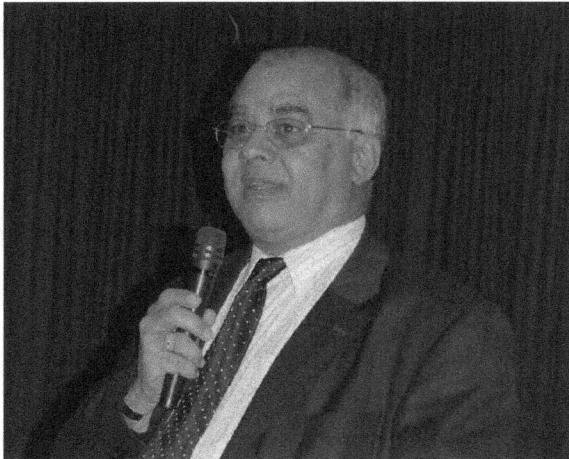

He met the love of his life Madeleine in Mauritius and married her on May 2, 1977. They migrated to Australia in 1982 and lived in Sydney in New South Wales, Mildura and Rosedale in country Victoria, and Carrum Downs in Melbourne.

Clancy has occupied various high level positions in Local Government Engineering and still practises his profession as a Municipal Engineer with the City of Greater Dandenong in Melbourne.

Madeleine and Clancy jointly took the initiative in 1994, to establish the very first web sites promoting Mauritius and its Cuisine. The 'Mauritius Australia Connection' and 'Recipes from Mauritius' web sites receive in excess of 4500 visits daily.

Both Madeleine and Clancy Philippe have contributed to numerous articles in magazines and travel guides on Mauritian Cuisine. They have travelled Australia extensively and went on a worldwide travel tour in 2007.

On February 11, 2011, Clancy lost Madeleine after a five year battle with breast and ovarian cancers. Other than work, he has since devoted himself to enjoying the love and company of his family, the Mauritius Australia Connection web site and writing about Madeleine and Mauritian Cuisine.

Mauritius Australia Connection http://www.cjp.net
Twitter: @ClancyP   Email: clancy@cjp.net
Facebook: http://www.facebook.com/clancy.philippe
Skype: clancy46
You can light a candle on Madeleine's Memorial web site at:
http://www.ilasting.com/madeleinephilippe.php

References

Servan-Schreiber, D., MD, PhD, *"Anti Cancer - A New Way of Life"*, 2008.

Agostini, M., - *"The Dying Experience and Learning How to Live"*.

Legge, K., - *"Weekend Australian Magazine Cover Story "The Death Whisperers"*, May 21, 2011.

Dr Barbato, M., *"Reflections of a Setting Sun" Healing Experiences around Death."*

Dr Barbato, M., *"Email dated August 20, 2011 to Clancy."*

Mauritius Australia Connection, *"Soul Mates, Spiritual Happiness and Family Love"* section on *'Soul Mates, Marriage in Heaven'* at http://www.cjp.net

Philippe, M., *Recipes from Mauritius* by Madeleine Philippe – http://ile-maurice.tripod.com

Noë, M.L., Poem - *"Je t'embrasse, fort. Très fort."*

Alfred, I., Poem – *"Let us celebrate Madeleine."*

Ducasse, E., *"Email dated March 9, 2011 to Clancy."*

Dallas, M., *"Emails dated February 9, 2011 and February 18, 2011 to Clancy."*

Haines, I., *"Note dated March 18, 2011 to Clancy and family."*

The author gratefully acknowledges permission to reproduce the following copyright material:

Legge, K., - *"Weekend Australian Magazine Cover Story "The Death Whisperers"*, May 21, 2011.

Dr Barbato, M., *"Reflections of a Setting Sun"Healing Experiences around Death, 2002.*

www.ingramcontent.com/pod-product-compliance
Lightning Source LLC
Chambersburg PA
CBHW060034030426
42334CB00019B/2321